PHYSICIAN
SUICIDE

CASES AND
COMMENTARIES

PHYSICIAN SUICIDE

CASES AND COMMENTARIES

Peter Yellowlees, MBBS, M.D.

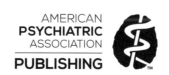

AMERICAN
PSYCHIATRIC
ASSOCIATION
PUBLISHING

If you wish to buy 50 or more copies of the same title, please go to www.appi.org/specialdiscounts for more information.

Copyright © 2019 American Psychiatric Association Publishing
ALL RIGHTS RESERVED
First Edition
Manufactured in the United States of America on acid-free paper

22 21 20 19 18   5 4 3 2 1

American Psychiatric Association Publishing
800 Maine Avenue, S.W., Suite 900
Washington, DC 20024-2812
www.appi.org

Library of Congress Cataloging-in-Publication Data
Names: Yellowlees, Peter, author. | American Psychiatric Association
   Publishing, publisher.
Title: Physician suicide : cases and commentaries / Peter Yellowlees.
Description: First edition. | Washington, D.C. : American Psychiatric Association
   Publishing, [2019] | Includes bibliographical references and index.
Identifiers: LCCN 2018016456 (print) | LCCN 2018017008 (ebook) | ISBN
   9781615372133 (ebook) | ISBN 9781615371693 (paperback : alk. paper)
Subjects: | MESH: Suicide—prevention & control | Physicians—psychology |
   Suicide—psychology | Burnout, Professional—therapy | Substance-Related
   Disorders—therapy | Case Reports
Classification: LCC R690 (ebook) | LCC R690 (print) | NLM WM 165 |
   DDC 610.69/5019—dc23
LC record available at https://lccn.loc.gov/2018016456

British Library Cataloguing in Publication Data
A CIP record is available from the British Library.

This book is dedicated to all the physicians whom I have treated as my patients over the past few decades in both Australia and the United States. They have taught me so much about the profession of medicine, and what an honor it is to practice in this most meaningful occupation.

Contents

About the Author

PETER YELLOWLEES, MBBS, M.D., is Professor of Psychiatry and Vice Chair for Faculty Development in the Department of Psychiatry at UC Davis School of Medicine in Sacramento, California. He is President of the American Telemedicine Association. After completing his medical training in London, Dr. Yellowlees worked in Australia for 20 years, where he completed his research doctorate at Flinders University and became chair of the department of psychiatry at the University of Queensland, before moving to the University of California, Davis, to continue his research in 2004. He has an international reputation in telemedicine and long-distance health and education delivery, and has for many years treated physicians as patients. Dr. Yellowlees has worked in public and private sectors, in academia, and in rural settings. He has published five books and more than 200 scientific articles and book chapters, and has been the author and video presenter of the internationally viewed "Medscape Psychiatry Minute" since 2009. He has been regularly involved in media presentations and has consulted to governments and private sector companies in several countries.

Preface

AS A PSYCHIATRIST I have been treating physicians with psychiatric and substance- and behavior-related illnesses for most of my career. A proportion of them have been suicidal, or contemplating suicide, as the ultimate form of self-harm and recrimination. As a human race we've long understood the importance of preventive maintenance for our cars, so it's odd that the importance of maintaining physician well-being is only now beginning to be widely recognized. Doctors who are sick are distressed by their illness, as are their families, and, if impaired, are more likely to make clinical mistakes and adversely affect the safety of their patients. There are many reasons why physicians don't maintain their health and well-being— including personal, professional, and systemic reasons—as well as many unintended consequences related to their practice environment that need to be addressed in order to facilitate their overall well-being. So what needs to happen, and why did I decide to write this book?

As an academic the answer is simple. I've learned a lot from my physician patients over many years, and I would like to impart that learning, not only to physicians but also to the general public, so that all can better understand the vagaries of the profession of medicine and, in this case, get inside the minds of physicians and recognize the unintended consequences of a professional workforce under stress.

Working with physicians as patients has been a constant learning process for me, and it has been a humbling and, at times, distressing process. I will never forget the two individual physicians whom I knew well and treated to the best of my ability who ultimately died by suicide. The large number of physician suicides—400 per year in the United States and many more around the world—is an utter tragedy, especially because many are preventable. So what have I learned? I know that when physicians talk about suicide, it's necessary to take them very seriously because, not surprisingly, they tend to be successful at this, as in most other things they attempt in life. I have learned never to assume that physicians know much about psychiatric conditions, because most physicians have little training in this area. I treat a physician patient in exactly the same manner that I would treat an intelligent nonphysician patient. There is no education program as to how to become a "doctor's doctor," so every doctor who has to take on other physicians as patients has to learn skills required to understand how best to treat colleagues successfully, noting that most physician patients are highly professional, respectful, humble, and grateful but may on occasion be intimidating, demanding, and challenging. There are few programs to teach physicians themselves the importance of self-care and a balanced lifestyle, although some such programs are starting to be available for residents. Equally, I've learned that physicians tend to be afraid to approach colleagues showing signs of distress, even though responding to a colleague's distress is a skill that can be learned and implemented. I've also learned that the professional culture of medicine, while it has many very positive aspects, counterintuitively has negative impacts on physicians' health and well-being and that parts of this professional culture, while hard to change, need to change. Today's millennial generation is starting to make some moves in that direction and seems to recognize the importance of the unintended consequences of the traditional physician lifestyle. The question is, will the rest of the profession listen and then effect change, or will such "change" be in name only, as so frequently happens in a conservative profession like medicine?

As someone who loves teaching, I know that cases and clinical studies are what students remember. Students can always go and look up the numeric facts and data after a lecture, but what brings a teacher's content to life is case studies and examples. Whenever I lecture I always start with clinical examples of the topic under discussion to serve as a "hook" for my students or audience. This gets them involved and makes them think of themselves and how they might relate to a character or respond in a given situation. In other words, it makes the topic more personal. In this book I have taken exactly the same approach and have written each chapter with a focus on a single case, which is then followed by a commentary explaining and highlighting certain aspects of the clinical case example. This is not a conventional way to write an educational book, but I believe it's an approach that will more effectively highlight some of the stressors affecting physicians than any conventional textbook could. My cases are fictional, however. They are not real, and so I have not had to seek permission from any patients, but they are all realistic and are examples of the sort of patients and situations I have encountered during many years of practice.

In writing these cases, I have thought and written like a novelist, creating people, situations, and events that are realistic but fiction. Inevitably some components of the content of some of the cases are derived from the stories of patients I have seen over the years, with the specifics heavily altered such that the situations are, I hope, completely unrecognizable. Other parts of the content have come from newspaper and media clippings, and several situations have been stimulated by stories appearing in the nonprint media or on the Internet. Some parts of the cases have appeared in legal documents published by medical boards and similar regulatory authorities around the world. Yet other parts of the cases are similar to those that have been mentioned by colleagues at conferences or in personal discussions, and other histories I've simply invented. I've tried hard to make sure that not a single one of my 10 "cases" is identifiable in any way with any patient whom I have ever seen. I've deliberately mixed and matched ideas and events and used my imagination to create the cases. My aim has always been to make the cases realistic, but not in any way identifiable or based on any single person. I hope that no patients whom I have ever seen will be able to recognize themselves, and if they believe they do, I can only say that such resemblance is completely accidental and likely related to my own unconscious and hidden memories. I believe that the 10 cases are realistic, but not real, and I hope that they ring true as examples of the sorts of lives that physicians lead and of the events that happen to them.

The case studies are written to bring the topic of physician suicide, and physician health, to life, and I hope, in particular, that readers from the lay community will appreciate the stresses and pressures that physicians face in practicing their profession. The commentaries in each chapter, on the other hand, are designed to enable this book to be used as a textbook by anyone who wishes to be a student of this topic. Here, rather than being a novelist, I have put on my academic hat to attempt to explain and discuss what I believe are the important elements of each case, allowing me over the course of the book to literally create a case-based curriculum on physician health and suicidal behaviors. As such, I believe that the cases could be used for small groups engaged in "case-based learning" on the topic of physician health. The book is not written in a random or accidental fashion, and the chapters build on one another so that readers, if they wish, may gradually learn many of the important things that I've learned over years of both treating and teaching physicians.

I've written *Physician Suicide* in a way that allows readers to read either the entire book sequentially from start to finish or individual chapters, all of which have specific foci and stand alone. Chapters 1–7 cover the full curriculum of physician health, ranging from professional lifestyle and expectations to burnout, through depression, anxiety, addictions, personality disorders, and aging, with a particular focus on the many interactions with suicide and suicidal behavior. Chapters 8–10 are much more focused on solutions—both treatment- and prevention-based, and individual and organizational—to these diverse problems.

Chapter 1 begins with one of several cases in the book of a completed physician suicide. The case is set during the funeral of a popular well-loved physician who struggled with depression and alcohol abuse. The commentary in this chapter concentrates on some of the core professional beliefs that drive physician practice and behavior and then moves on to the epidemiology and clinical issues surrounding suicidality in physicians and the impact of a physician suicide on treating providers, as well as the potential preventive effect of screening for alcohol and drugs within the medical profession. In Chapter 2, I move this discussion forward by exploring the linkage with burnout and how this condition may lead to depression and suicidal ideation. I also address how burnout may be reduced by organizational and individual factors, such as enabling shared collaborative decision making and building individual resilience. Chapter 3 focuses on responses by other physicians and health workers to a physician suicide and ways to screen and engage physicians in treatment; in the process, I take a dynamic look at the development of professionalism in physicians and discuss why the impact of delayed gratification is so important, and potentially problematic, throughout their lives. Chapter 4 is primarily about the treatment of alcohol abuse and addiction and its relationship with suicidality but introduces the topic of telemedicine and health technologies, and how they can improve current treatment and protect individual physicians' privacy to allow them to access confidential treatment. In this chapter I also discuss the reasons that many physicians do not receive the best possible evidence-based treatments for alcohol use disorders, such as medication-assisted treatments. In Chapter 5, I address narcotic abuse, self-prescribing, and barriers to care for physicians, especially physicians' often realistic fear of regulatory responses and loss of their medical license. I also highlight the success of physician health programs in monitoring the treatment of physician addicts. In Chapter 6, I move on to discuss the difficult challenge of how to manage and treat physicians who are disruptive and have severe personality disorders, and to explore why the healthcare profession has been so tolerant of such destructive individuals for so many years. In Chapter 7, which completes the group of clinical issues that primarily affect physicians, I focus on elderly physicians and their reluctance to retire, the impact nationally of the aging physician workforce, and the difficulty obtaining and undertaking high-quality fitness-for-duty assessments that correctly identify which elderly doctors are cognitively impaired and which are not.

In Chapter 8, I focus on the clinical treatment by physicians of physicians and some of the potential boundary and professional concerns raised, as well as address gender and cross-cultural issues and the reasons that female doctors are substantially more at risk of suicide than their age- and gender-matched community nonphysicians when they have disorders such as bipolar disorder or depression. Chapters 9 and 10 are primarily about solutions to the problems of physician health. In Chapter 9, I examine the processes and effectiveness of formal physician health programs and well-being committees, noting that many doctors in small private practices are much less likely to be able to access these programs. In Chapter 10, I look at the need for professional culture change and preventive and lifestyle solutions for individual physicians, as well as the need for better organizational management of clinical workflows and workloads, which are all too often driven by administrative requirements or the introduction of innovative practice technologies such as electronic records in the physician workplace.

This book is intended to be read by any physician and medical or premedical students, as well as by members of the general public, in the hope that it will highlight the professional mind-set of most physicians and the ways in which this mind-set interacts with some of the stressors and illnesses that affect physicians, and therefore potentially their patients. More importantly, I hope this book describes the many pathways that can be taken to both prevent the tragedy of physician suicide and reduce the impact of the related disorders that can lead to this tragic outcome. Having been a practicing physician myself for many years, I know that the profession of medicine is one of the most meaningful and important careers that it's possible for an individual to embark on. Today's medical students and residents are wonderful, intelligent, and committed people, and hopefully they will not be as afflicted as previous generations by the tragedy of suicide and the range of other disorders described in this book. The medical profession needs to take serious steps to improve physician health and thereby reduce the number of physicians who kill themselves each year.

Peter Yellowlees, MBBS, M.D.
Sacramento, California
March 2018

Acknowledgments

I'VE THOUGHT ABOUT WRITING this book for several years and wish to acknowledge primarily the interest of my wife, Barb, and her support throughout this process. She not only has made a major contribution to the writing of the book as my primary editor and literary critic, but also has listened to me and critiqued my ideas as I struggled to constantly improve the fictional cases I've included, ensuring that they remained both realistic and relevant.

There is little mention in the literature on physician health of the details of the daily events and pressures that contribute to the lifestyle of many physicians and that may have some unintended consequences, of which suicide is the most extreme. This book is an attempt to document the pain and suffering that physicians are trained to deny, especially in front of their patients, in the hope that it may improve the understanding of the lives of current generations of physicians and prevent further suffering in future generations and their loved ones.

I have been heavily influenced in developing the style of this book by Oliver Sacks, who wrote a series of articles that were eventually turned into the best-selling book *The Man Who Mistook His Wife for a Hat and Other Clinical Tales* (New York, Summit Books, 1985). Sacks wrote about real patients he had treated in each chapter of his book, and then discussed their disorders from a neurological perspective. I have modeled the style of this book on his work, but with the major difference that, while he discussed real patients, mine are fictional.

I have worked with numerous dedicated people in the area of physician health during the past decade at the University of California, Davis (UC Davis), and wish to acknowledge all of them, whether they are mentioned by name here or not, as well as all of my many physician patients. My departmental chair, Robert Hales, M.D., has always been very supportive of this interest, as has the team from the UC Davis Office of Medical Administration, including Alan Siefkin, M.D., James Kirk, M.D., Leslie Navarra, and Mija Ryer in association with their other support staff, and Ann Madden Rice and Colleen Clancy, Ph.D., also at UC Davis. I have worked with numerous faculty on the Medical Staff Well-Being Committee at UC Davis over the past 8 years and wish especially to acknowledge Margaret Rea, Ph.D., Andres Sciolla, M.D., Jessica Haskins, Ph.D., Celia Chang, M.D., Daniel Link, M.D., Carol Kirshnit, Ph.D., Debra Kahn, M.D., Katren Tyler, Nasim Hedayati, M.D., and Jeffrey Uppington, M.D.

Individuals who have helped me with collegiality, advice, and assistance as I've continuously learned about the many aspects of physician health from outside California include Jay Shore, M.D., Michael Gendel, M.D., and Doris Gunderson, M.D. Within California I wish to acknowledge the leadership shown in this area by Michael Parr, M.D., and the members of California Public Protection and Physician Health, especially Gail Jara and Karen Miotto, M.D., and locally by the Sacramento Sierra Valley Medical Society, particularly Aileen Wetzel and Rajiv Misquitta, M.D. Finally, many expert papers and books are quoted and referenced throughout this book, and I thank all of these contributors who are so referenced.

CHAPTER

1

Personal Stress Therapy

IT WAS A BEAUTIFUL SPRING DAY, blue sky and bright sun, as I entered the back of the church for the funeral of one of my patients—a physician I had treated for the last 3 years. I was diffident about attending and took a place in an empty pew near the back where I could be present for the service and pay my last respects to Dr. Marco Bianchi.

As Marco's psychiatrist I felt the weight of sadness at his passing and wondered if I could have done anything else to prevent his death. Would hospitalization have made a difference? Would any other combination of antidepressants have been more effective? Should we have focused more on psychotherapy, and were there dynamic issues that I didn't address with him? Should I have followed him up more assertively in the weeks prior to his death? Could I have engaged his wife and children in more therapy sessions to change the outcome? So many questions had been going through my head since I learned of his suicide a week before. Yet I knew that despite my efforts, Marco had stopped coming to appointments and had not been returning my calls for the past 6 weeks. Should I have cer-

1

tified him and had him hospitalized against his will? Would it have made a difference? I had discussed hospitalization with him several times over the years, but Marco remained completely against it. He felt it would not help him and that it could put his medical license at risk. I took his concern to keep his physician license intact as a sign that he was not planning on killing himself, however depressed and hopeless he felt, because at least he still had an eye for his future. In the end, even the personal and professional pride he took in being a physician was not enough to keep Marco going. Although it seemed logical that I had done all that I could, I struggled with a sense of failure and self-questioning. I hoped that coming to his funeral would let me think about him peacefully, to start to resolve my own personal loss, and to say good-bye to a patient whom I had known well for years. Marco had originally chosen me as his doctor because he had found out that I treated many other physicians for their psychiatric and substance-related disorders, but little did I know that he would be the first of my physician patients to complete his own suicide.

I settled in at the back of the church and started to read through the funeral pamphlet. A photo of Marco taken probably a decade previously adorned the front cover. As I surveyed the chosen hymns and quietly read through the comforting 23rd psalm, printed in full on the second page, I started to relax. I looked up and to my surprise I saw Marco's wife, Theresa, whom I knew well from many joint sessions with her husband, quietly walking up the aisle toward me. She had her brown hair up in a bun and was wearing a simple black suit and heels. Her only piece of jewelry was a gold wedding ring on her left finger. Her face could not hide her exhaustion and the strain of the solemn event that day. She tipped her head toward me, indicating that she wanted me to follow her down the aisle to join her grieving Italian family seated at the front of the church. I followed her toward the front, passing Dr. Bianchi's coffin on the way. It felt strange walking beside the closed coffin that held the remains of Marco, my patient. As I approached the family I couldn't help noticing the many tearful and red eyes, especially among the children, and their communal feel of deep sadness and loss.

I sat down where Theresa indicated, in a pew behind the family, a few yards from Dr. Bianchi's coffin. A beautiful carved mahogany container covered in a massive arrangement of white roses within which lay the body of an eminent physician, loved and respected by many in his family and community—a man who was externally successful but who, as I and his wife knew only too well, had struggled all his career to fight his own demons, sometimes successfully, who, ultimately, in his mid-fifties, had surrendered in the battle to survive.

The service commenced. A Catholic mass in a now crowded church. A family, a community in mourning showing its distress and, among many, their shock at the unexpected death. I wondered how they would manage the fact that Marco had died by suicide and how they would acknowledge this. Or would they? And who, if any, in this gathering really knew what had happened to him?

The eulogies were heartfelt. Marco's son told of his father's love and sensitivity to his children; of his career in medicine and his commitment to his patients, often putting their concerns ahead of his own needs; and of his work as an emergency physician that had led to him volunteering overseas and helping a number of charitable organizations during his career. His daughter told stories from her childhood of camping trips, family movie nights, and her father's love of adventure. Many from the community told stories of Marco helping out neighbors and always seeming friendly and outgoing. Colleagues from his workplace spoke more about happier times with Marco in the early years. His wife, whom he was separated from at the time of his death, sat quietly and listened. No one mentioned the cause of his death, although all agreed the abrupt and early nature of his departure was a tragedy. As I listened to the loving remembrances of Dr. Bianchi's life, I reflected that I had heard similar stories from his perspective during our many sessions together. This man who loved being a physician had been respected and loved by his family and friends and his community.

I remembered the first time I met Dr. Bianchi 3 years before. He had been referred to me by a colleague, Dr. Sarter, who worked at the same hospital and who thought Marco might be depressed, as he was having difficulty keeping up with his work and seemed more irritated and easily upset than usual.

Marco was memorable from the start, arriving 20 minutes late with the usual doctor's excuse of a patient phone call. He was instantly charismatic—tall, dark, and slim—although with a worn and rather crumpled tired appearance, looking older than his documented age. No sign of the initial anxiety that most patients showed when meeting a psychiatrist for the first time. He spoke in a smooth, deep, and slightly accented voice, immediately giving me the impression he could have been sent from central casting to play the role of an Italian gentleman scholar.

"I'm really only here to satisfy Dr. Sarter. He's a nice man. He means well and is concerned about me, but I think we can get this session over quickly and then I'll reassure him all is fine with me. I've had a number of problems in the past, but they are all behind me now, and I just wish I hadn't mentioned anything about them to Dr. Sarter."

"What sort of problems?" I asked.

He looked somewhat defensive. "I don't think we need go into much detail. I had to stop practice for a few months when I was a junior attending and went into detox. You know, one of those drug and alcohol programs for doctors where they monitor you for a few years afterwards. I did a 12-step program and went into regular counseling. I did great and was sober for years afterwards."

He stopped speaking and looked at me carefully before continuing. "I'm sure all the doctors you see say the same. I started drinking heavily at frat parties in college and continued in medical school. It was all just the usual culture—we worked hard and played hard. We celebrated all our exam successes, and if things weren't so good, we drowned our sorrows. Alcohol became a big part of my life."

He continued: "And in residency we continued the same way, although with all the shifts we did in my training as an emergency physician, I added in sleeping pills so that I could get some sleep at odd hours when I wasn't at work. I know a number of my friends did the same. We even used to compare which meds were most effective, especially when we were on night shift and had to sleep during the day. I guess it all just steamrollered from there—by the time I was through residency and working as a specialist I was keeping myself going on a combination of alcohol and sleeping pills. I eventually added narcotics, because they were so easily available at work and I felt I could manage these drugs as something I could use occasionally. Unfortunately, occasional became routine, and I began to get into difficulties at home and at work. Anyway, that's all behind me now, so is there anything else you want to know, because I haven't got a great deal of time today and have to get going soon? My shift in the emergency room starts in an hour and I can't keep my patients waiting."

As I sat and listened to the eulogies and the rest of the service, I thought about the remainder of that first noteworthy session I had spent with him. He told me I was the first psychiatrist he had consulted for over 15 years because he had decided that he could "beat" the substance problem himself. After 5 years of sobriety in his thirties, he had stopped seeing a counselor and also quit attending Alcoholics Anonymous. I remembered him starting to tell me about life after that.

"Life has been difficult at times. My marriage has been problematic for years. I know I work too hard and my wife is always complaining that she's the third part of my life, behind work and what I believe is my controlled drinking, although she disagrees. She has left me a couple of times briefly, but she knows I love our children and she wants to keep the family together, so she has come back each time when I have promised to see someone. In fact, that's the real reason I'm here today—she told me I have to get treatment or she won't return this time. This is the first time she has actually threatened divorce. I know I'm not a perfect husband in any way and that my drinking has caused problems between us. But the fact remains that I love her, and I know she loves me."

Dr. Bianchi's story continued emerging slowly and in staccato style during that first and many subsequent sessions. He frequently denied and intellectualized his problems—blaming others for his family and personal misfortunes and difficulties, while minimizing what sounded like major problems in his personal life that were at least partially related to his drinking. He referred to his excessive drinking as his "personal stress therapy," often shortening this to a typical medical jargon acronym, "PST," as a way of denying its significance and not having to admit that he was an alcoholic. He was always anxious to discuss his successes and his ability to keep his professional life going reasonably well, and I became used to his defensive and sometimes boastful style of conversation whereby he consistently minimized any problems he was having at home or work. I remembered him pulling out a copy of his résumé from his briefcase and showing me that he had published over 50 peer-reviewed scientific articles and had lectured in several countries. This was something that I heard several of the speakers at the funeral comment on, as well as the fact that he was the first person in his large immigrant Italian family not only to attend medical school but to graduate from college.

The last of the speakers, a lifelong friend, was the one who described him best, and brought me back to the present, and the funeral.

"Marco was a lifelong friend of mine. He was someone who gave to us all. He gave of himself to his friends, his children, and his community, and in particular to his work. He was very aware of succeeding in all that he did and found it very hard to admit any problems. He enjoyed being with people but found it hard to be intimate—he always seemed to feel he was a physician first and a person second. As such he did have difficulties. The fact that he died so young and suddenly, and that we are all here at his funeral, way too early in his life, is proof of that. His wife, Theresa, who has been with him for over 25 years, knows this only too well, as do some of his friends who have had to help him on occasions. We know that he was tortured at times and can only imagine how he felt at the end. Such an outgoing, gregarious, and generous friend, whom we loved, and who loved us all, died alone, preferring not to ask for the sort of help that he would have given to any of us. His death is such a tragedy. He was so confident that he could manage his own problems that he would not let us help him, even when we reached out. We'll always remember him. He is in heaven now.

At peace finally, but with his sense of caring, he'll probably soon be doing good works for the angels. I just hope that he looks after himself more in the next life than he did in this."

After the funeral Theresa moved through the crowd to find me. She had attended numerous sessions with Marco to see me and had tried to persuade and cajole him to maintain sobriety and stop his polysubstance abuse. Today her voice was shaky, and it took a few minutes for her to compose herself. She asked me to sit with her for a few minutes so she could talk to me and thank me. I had not expected this from her, especially at this point in time. She talked about Marco's great suffering for many years but told me that he was grateful for the counseling and support I had given to him and that at times he thought he could see a light at the end of his long tunnel. She said Marco had greatly valued his relationship with me and that she was grateful for my attempts to help him. She knew Marco was his own worst enemy and that somehow what had happened was not a surprise. She pointed out that although Marco had the support he needed, he alone chose to end his own life, and had done so on his own terms, making sure he would not be found. She said she was in part relieved that Marco's suffering was over but also concerned that she and the children would have to deal with this unhappy ending for the rest of their lives. She was worried about the long-term impact on her children.

As I left the church I couldn't help but wonder if there was anything I could have done differently to alter the course for Marco. What had happened in the past, and why was I questioning my efforts to help him?

Marco had agreed to continue meeting regularly with me after our first encounter. Throughout our early sessions he remained defensive and irritated, with his anger and frustration at himself often directed externally.

"I really don't need to be seeing you. I don't know why my drinking is being seen as a problem. It has never interfered with my work except when I had to go to detox years ago."

I tried to use motivational interviewing techniques with him, whereby I attempted to define exactly what level of insight into his drinking he had, and what amount of change he could tolerate or was prepared to commit to. Sadly, I had little success with these approaches and numerous others.

"But why do you think you drink so much, and why do you see this as your 'therapy'? Why your 'PST'? Not everyone in your situation does this. What would it take to make you stop drinking? Would you be prepared to set yourself a maximum number of drinks per week, and keep to it, or perhaps even to quit completely?"

In the early months of our relationship he seemed poorly motivated to stop drinking. "There's no reason to stop. I like it. I'm used to it. I have always let off steam in this way. I'm not alcoholic or anything like that. If I chose to I could always stop for a few days. I just don't want to. When I feel down, it actually makes me feel better. I like my PST. It's my friend. I'm less depressed when I have a drink or two and worry less about all the issues I have to deal with. It helps me blot out the things Theresa says to me. I cannot stand her nagging me, even though I know she's trying to help. Let's face it, I could take all sorts of other drugs if I wanted to—it's easy for me to get hold of tranquilizers or narcotics in my line of work. I could be writing my own prescriptions easily enough. So surely having a few drinks is not too bad an alternative?"

As I got to know Marco better over the first few sessions it became apparent that his drinking was only part of his problem and that he was also significantly depressed but trying to hide this. He had a family characterized by high rates of both alcohol abuse and depression, with his father, two cousins, and several distant relations affected by one or the other disease, or both, and one cousin who had died by suicide in his early twenties. He described a history of recurrent severe depression, first in medical school, at which time he was prescribed antidepressants, then following his forced detox in his early thirties, when he also took medications for a couple of years. He became increasingly focused on describing his depression, often as an excuse to avoid talking about his alcohol intake.

"It's like carrying a 50-pound backpack all day. I just feel completely exhausted. My mind won't work as fast as it usually does, and I can't remember details like I should. It can be embarrassing at work when I forget the name or details of a key drug or of a patient that I should know and have to stop and think. Usually I would know all that sort of stuff instantly. I notice that my sleep is poor and I don't handle shifts so easily. I even see that my academic work goes down, and I find it harder than usual to finish writing my papers or preparing lectures for students and residents."

"How often does this happen?" I asked.

"I've had maybe five or six such episodes during my life—usually for about 6 months, but in several instances for longer than that. I ended up taking 3 months off during medical school, during which I was treated with therapy and antidepressants. I even thought of suicide as being a way out of my troubles, but I never tried it, and I wouldn't ever do that now because I know how it would hurt Theresa and the kids. In my thirties I guess I was a sort of "dry drunk" when I was maintaining my sobriety after my first medical board report for a DUI and the required treatment and monitoring. Being a dry drunk is like feeling depressed, only you blame it on the lack of alcohol and just want to get back to drinking to improve your mood. I craved alcohol every day. I hated that process, which lasted for 5 years. I had to have random weekly urine alcohol screens to prove I was sober and fit to work, but I managed it with the help of the antidepressants prescribed by my addiction specialist. What he didn't know was that I was also taking sleeping pills and tranquilizers that I was able to self-prescribe, to get through work, and that they made me feel better, so I didn't miss the alcohol as much. Lucky they didn't test for those."

It became apparent early on in my treatment of Dr. Bianchi that he was going to be very difficult to treat and that he was proud of his ability to deceive his previous doctors. He had been abusing alcohol and prescription drugs since early medical school and had never been sober from either for any length of time except for during hospital detoxification, which lasted for 3 months. More worrying was the strong history of depression, and his linkage of these symptoms with alcohol and tranquilizers as "therapy" for the depression. He had only moderate insight into his situation and had never had therapy in any formal way. He had substantial long-term marital problems despite his tolerant and supportive but rather dependent wife, whom he admitted he treated badly. Despite all of this, his core love, that of being a physician, was still intact, and he gained tremendous strength through his interactions with his patients and through his persona and role as a physician within his close-knit Italian community.

We spent some time after a few sessions negotiating a treatment plan, including medication and individual and marital therapy, and I focused on his denial and intellectualization, the major psychological defenses that allowed him to avoid insight and treatment.

I particularly remembered his frequent attempts to reassure me about his health and his resilience. "I don't know why you're so worried about me. I have been coping fine for the past 30 years and have just gained promotion once again at work. I'm able to control my drinking, and now that you have me on my antidepressants again, I don't need any extra tranquilizers. My work is going great. My kids are through school, and I just need to start spending more time with Theresa so that we can work things out and get on better together."

He frequently tried to minimize the importance of his treatment, telling me with a sense of inflated self-importance: "Why, isn't it ridiculous that I, as an internationally known emergency physician, am coming to see a psychiatrist to get the sort of advice that anyone could give? You would think I would be able to look after myself fine. After all, I know about all this stuff and studied it in medical school." However, he kept coming to all the sessions, despite his objections related to his self-perceived feeling of failure to manage himself, and the consequent stigma of needing to see a psychiatrist, and I regularly met with him at least once or twice per month.

Over the next 3 years I saw him jointly with Theresa on numerous occasions. I was concerned that he refused to go to see a therapist for marital counseling despite repeated requests from his wife. These sessions were frequently difficult and painful for both of them. Marco would often end up in tears as he confronted the pain he was causing his wife and children, while Theresa, with some prodding from me, was gradually able to be more assertive, threatening to leave him several times. Gradually Marco attempted to reduce and then stop drinking with the help of medication-assisted treatment that I prescribed. This included a variety of antidepressants and mood stabilizers, as well as anticraving drugs. Finally, he achieved 6 months of sobriety with the help of voluntary random monitoring of his urine and regular attendance at AA meetings for health professionals, where he felt his fellow members could understand him better than his family or myself.

He sometimes tried to teach me my business. "You know, I think you should start some support groups for your patients. You could have them here, and I could help you run them. I could become a group leader. You can't believe how awkward some of the group members are. They really need more guidance and direction. That's something you might be able to do better, instead of just sitting there and seeing lots of individual patients like me. These are people who are not going to change a great deal with individual therapy alone, especially from someone who hasn't been through what they've been through and therefore can't really understand." His arrogance and denial still shone through on occasions, but despite this, I began to be more hopeful of his success, as he and his wife seemed to be communicating somewhat better and he was maintaining his sobriety, which I routinely checked with random drug screens. Unfortunately, I was eventually proven wrong.

I had been seeing Marco fairly regularly in the year before his death, but then he began missing appointments with me, which was unlike him. He seemed cagey and wary on the phone when I called and said he was going to take a break from our sessions for a while. I tried to persuade him otherwise but with no success. I was very concerned and called Theresa to see if she could persuade him to reengage with me. She told me she had moved out and had given Marco an ultimatum that she would divorce him if he couldn't stop drinking. She agreed to speak to him but was unable to persuade him to continue his regular appointments with me.

Knowing how depressed he could become, I was very concerned for his safety, so I took the unusual step of phoning the police and asking them to go and visit him at his home to do a welfare safety check. Two police met with him at his home. He apparently presented well. Somewhat aggrieved and hostile initially, he was able to convince them that he was not an immediate danger to himself. He was always so good at holding himself together for up to an hour at a time, seemingly rational and not a danger to himself or others. So despite my concerns, the visiting police were unable to write a hold on him and force him into a psychiatric hospital, which in retrospect could have possibly saved his life.

Marco died by suicide 6 weeks after our last appointment. It seems that during this time he and Theresa had had several significant arguments. He had returned to drinking heavily, especially once he moved out of their home, and took 3 weeks off from work, ostensibly to have a vacation, but actually to stay at home and drink.

A week before his death Marco appeared at work one day obviously inebriated, smelling of alcohol and clearly unfit to work in the emergency department. His departmental chairman was urgently called to see him and found him angry, belligerent, and partially intoxicated, admitting to drinking alcohol and taking tranquilizers before coming into work. His chairman, not surprisingly, sent him home and put him on immediate administrative leave, a public process that occurred in front of all the staff in the emergency department and that Marco, not surprisingly, found completely humiliating. A doctor being taken off duty "for cause" is an event that is always a potential precursor to being reported to the state medical board. Given his past history of similar behavior many years ago, he would have realized this was likely to be very serious and might eventually lead to his having his medical license revoked. At the very best he was heading for a detox admission and would be required to start the treatment process that in the past had led to sobriety for a number of years. He would have known that this time around the process would be much tighter and would not allow him to continue taking tranquilizers. His professional life, including his reputation, was all he really had left at this time, and this was now in jeopardy.

Unfortunately, Marco's departmental chair did not know he was seeing me, and Marco's pride may have made it impossible for him to call to me for help now that he had been found out; his secret was out in the open. I was not notified of these developments at the time. It appears that he went home and continued drinking heavily, and consuming many tranquilizers, over the next few days while planning his next, and final, step.

What was sure was that his professional knowledge made it certain that his suicide would be successful. He planned his death very carefully and took numerous precautions to make sure that his plan would not be interrupted. He booked a motel room for a weekend in a small country town about a hundred miles away from his home. He told no one about his plan and arrived early the following Friday evening, put a "do not disturb" notice on his door, and wrote a letter to his wife and children, which he signed and sealed and left beside his bed. He considerately and tragically left a separate note with his wife's phone number beside the letter so that she could be telephoned when he was found. In the letter to his family he wrote that he loved them and apologized for not having been a better husband and father. He finished by saying that he was exhausted and that they would no longer need to worry about him. He then took a carefully planned massive overdose of a variety of medications he had stolen from the emergency department, which he washed down with copious amounts of whiskey. He sat down in front of the television and watched Friday night football, continuing to drink as he gradually lost consciousness. He was found dead on Monday morning by a maid after he had failed to check out at the correct time.

Losing a patient in this way for a physician, especially a psychiatrist, is in itself one of the biggest losses it's possible to have. I know that I'll never forget Marco. I'll always wonder if I could have done anything different. If I might have somehow helped him more. Whether I could have prevented his suicide. The rational part of me says that all was done that could have been done. Certainly, being thanked by Theresa at his funeral reduced my feelings of guilt and self-doubt, but the impossibility of knowing whether Marco might still be alive today had I acted differently cannot be changed. It's a fact. It's a fact that I have learned to live with and will always live with.

Commentary

Marco's story is a tragedy, and one that is all too common. A highly trained emergency physician who in many ways was living the American dream, having succeeded professionally and gained the respect of his large Italian family and his community. From all outward perspectives he was an example of professional excellence and success with his family and community commitments, yet he struggled inwardly and ultimately succumbed, dying a lonely and isolated individual.

It is estimated that about 300–400 physicians die by suicide every year in the United States (Center et al. 2003). That is the equivalent of two large medical school classes. We do not know the exact numbers because formal coroner-reported statistics are certainly underestimated. Some suicides, such as those involving single-car accidents, do not end up being reported as suicides because of lack of evidence, and, at least in past years, some physician suicides are covered over by reporting colleagues because of the stigma involved. Each one of them is a tragedy, and all are associated with individual, family, and community pain and regret because no one ever wants to see, or hear of, a physician suicide.

The public does not think of physicians as being at risk of suicide. They are meant to display a kind of selfless professional immortality, certainly to their patients. It is always assumed that they are looking after themselves and are able to manage any illnesses they have (because they are only human of course) in a way that enables them to care properly for their patients. This philosophy is learned from an early stage at medical school and makes excellent sense in terms of a physician's patient care role. If, as a patient, you are sick yourself, then you hardly want to be treated by a sick doctor, so physicians learn to separate their own needs and difficulties from patients behind a professional veneer.

How does this happen? The first ethical rule of medicine that all physicians are taught is the Latin phrase *primum non nocere*, which translates to "first do no harm." This is of core relevance to the issue of physician health because impaired or suicidal physicians may well put their patients at risk as a result of their own illness. As a consequence of this, most medical boards, the groups that license and regulate physicians, are primarily set up to be consumer, or patient, protection agencies. Such agencies are not there to protect physicians. Rather, they protect patients by attempting to ensure that sick, incompetent, or impaired physicians are not able to practice in an unsafe or unsupervised manner. Physicians often find this hard to reconcile. They pay substantial annual fees to receive their medical licenses, yet paradoxically the licensing authority is not there primarily to protect them. As a result, being reported to the state medical board is very significant and a serious situation that can potentially lead to the loss of a medical license, livelihood, and self-esteem and to major financial and personal difficulties.

Marco turned up at work obviously intoxicated, and it was immediately realized that he was unfit to work. Who could imagine having a drunk doctor making potentially life-threatening decisions? What patient would want to be treated by such a physician? Not surprisingly Marco's most senior colleague was immediately called to investigate and assess his fitness to practice. Marco had already been reported to a medical board early in his career for having alcohol-related problems and had been treated in what is still frequently called a "diversion program," which exists in most U.S. states. The medical board had taken away his full medical license and had given him a probationary license for 5 years that was dependent on him entering an alcohol treatment and monitoring program and maintaining sobriety proved with random urine alcohol testing. In essence, he was allowed to practice, with some clinical supervision from a colleague, and had been "diverted" from losing his license completely. At the end of the 5-year period he was able to apply for a full license again and to begin normal unsupervised practice. There has been a lot of research looking at the effectiveness of these highly regulated monitoring and treatment programs, where the cost of failure (or lack of sobriety with a positive alcohol or drug screen) is high and involves giving up practice immediately. They are remarkably successful, with most such programs reporting that over 80% of physicians maintain sobriety and continue to practice medicine in their own specialty successfully at the 5-year mark (Rose et al. 2017). What we do not have is information about the long-term follow-up of these physicians and whether they, like Marco, tend to relapse and become unwell again in later years. Given that alcohol and substance use disorders are chronic remitting diseases, it is likely that a proportion of these physicians do relapse later in their careers, but it is unknown how large this proportion is.

Physicians, just like airline pilots, are put in a position of extreme trust by society, and the great majority of physicians and pilots meet the requirements of this trust given to them extremely well. But how can we trust those physicians who have the often lifelong diseases of alcohol or substance abuse to keep themselves safe and to never be intoxicated when treating their patients? Some have wondered whether we should be thinking about treating doctors more like airline pilots. No pilots are allowed to drink within 24 hours of flying and are routinely and randomly drug tested. Increasingly physicians are being drug tested, as are many other employees, when they start employment with a health system, but very few systems go beyond that to drug or alcohol testing physicians either routinely or randomly. Perhaps they should? What does happen widely is that many health systems have policies that stipulate that they can test a physician "for cause"—in other words, if something in the physician's behavior or presentation leads to suspicion of inappropriate substance use. But by the time a physician is demonstrating impaired behavior at work, it is frequently fairly late in his or her illness and the time for early intervention and prevention is past.

What about the many physicians who are self-employed or who work in small private group practices, which is where over 50% of all U.S. doctors practice? These professionals are beyond the reach of the policies of any health systems, and unless individual patients are concerned about them and report them to a medical board, there are many fewer potential checks affecting them, unless they choose to refer themselves to a statewide physician health program. Look at Marco as an example. Suppose he had been a cardiologist in a small private practice and had turned up at work drunk. He might have covered up his behavior much more easily than in a busy emergency department where there were many staff. In the clinic he could have possibly worked all day as his inebriation gradually reduced. Or more seriously, he could have continued drinking surreptitiously, perhaps taking vodka and chewing mints, and stayed intoxicated while working.

If Marco had always been employed in health systems where random urine testing was routine, he would have most likely had a much more successful life. His compulsive drinking, and his denial of his problem, would have been less likely to occur, and the whole direction and outcome of his life might have been changed. Of course, as an alternative to this situation, he might have deliberately changed his style of medical practice and worked in a system that was smaller and where such testing did not occur, hence allowing him to continue to drink. We shall never know, but this leaves us with important questions.

Should physicians be treated like pilots and be routinely and randomly drug tested at times that they cannot predict? And if so, for which drugs and for how long? Should someone like Marco have been put on a lifelong testing program at least while he was practicing medicine? And how do we tell whether physicians who test positive for, say, opiates such as codeine, or amphetamines such as Ritalin, are unfit to practice? Were these even their chosen drugs of abuse, or, like Marco, were they abusing other drugs unknown to their treating physicians? They may have a medical reason to be taking these drugs and may actually be much safer physicians when they are taking them than when not doing so. These issues should be explored.

Now that we've reviewed some of the professional underpinnings of medicine, with a focus on the unintended consequences for some physicians like Marco, for whom medicine was an excessive first love and major life focus, let's move on to the Hippocratic Oath, another core ethical component of medical practice.

There are many modernized variations of this ancient Greek oath. All physicians from all U.S. medical schools, when they attend their commencement ceremonies to graduate from medical school, literally stand up in front of the audience, made up of their families and friends. They then solemnly swear to live their professional lives in accord with an oath that is typically derived in some form or another from the original Greek version. Thankfully no one any longer swears the original oath, which assumed all physicians were male and which did not permit cutting patients in any way! Modern-day oaths are frequently written by the students themselves but are still usually derived from a number of adapted versions of the original. In these oaths the students typically pledge to put patients ahead of themselves, to always act in the best interests of their patients, and to not discriminate against any individual or group of patients based on gender, race, sexual orientation, or religion. These are without doubt very important principles to live and work by and for most physicians are congruent with their beliefs. Importantly, they have the underlying message that physicians are elevated to a higher level than others in their community because of their service to others ahead of themselves, and for people like Marco, this can make it much harder for them to seek help for themselves. After all, if you think and believe that you have a higher calling than all those whom you know, how are you going to ask them for help when you have your own needs?

We know that physicians find it very hard to ask for help when they are unwell. Marco was one of those individuals. He had gone many years treating himself only partially successfully before being referred to a psychiatrist by a colleague. Up to half of all physicians in the United States do not even have a primary care physician with whom they are registered. Physicians frequently end up treating themselves, and sometimes also their families, and often do both badly because they are unable to objectively view themselves and their problems, never mind do a proper physical or psychiatric examination on themselves or their family! So, while the Hippocratic Oath is an important ethical underpinning of much of medical practice, it does have an unfortunate unintended consequence of potentially leading doctors to be less able to seek care for themselves when they need it. Should this be changed? Or perhaps when medical student classes write their new versions of the oath, they should include in it a component that indicates that they also need to look after their own health so that they are fit to look after others. Think about the airline industry again as an example, where passengers are told to put on air masks first before assisting others such as children. This is what physicians need to learn to do and something that Marco just did not understand.

A related issue is the difficulty that physicians have in identifying a colleague who is at risk of suicide and then approaching them sensitively, as will be discussed in more detail in Chapters 3 and 8. If Marco's colleagues had been able to do this, then perhaps his suicide might have been avoided. The American Medical Association (AMA) (2018) has produced an excellent online module in their STEPS Forward series on preventing physician distress and suicide. In this module, they describe four steps to identify at-risk physicians within an organization and refer them to appropriate care:

1. Talk about the risk factors and warning signs for suicide.
2. Take steps to standardize care seeking in your organization.
3. Make it easy to find help.
4. Consider creating a support system for physicians in your organization.

Throughout this book there are examples of settings where these steps have, or have not, been implemented, with differing outcomes, and similarly in the AMA module there are a number of carefully written case scenarios that demonstrate the importance of the steps.

Despite this knowledge, and the increasingly frequent implementation of support systems for physicians, why did Marco see suicide as a "solution" to his problems, and why are physicians at more risk of suicide than nonphysicians (Center et al. 2003)? Let's examine what we know about this.

The American Foundation for Suicide Prevention (AFSP) (2018; www. afsp.org) has an excellent Web site that includes a good summary of facts about physician depression and suicide written by Christine Moutier, M.D., as follows[1]:

> Physicians have higher rates of burnout, depressive symptoms, and suicide risk than the general population. Physicians and trainees can experience high degrees of mental health distress and are less likely than other members of the public to seek mental health treatment. Physicians report several barriers to seeking mental health care, including time constraints, hesitancy to draw attention to self-perceived weakness, and concerns about reputation and confidentiality. Other facts include:
>
> - Suicide generally is caused by the convergence of multiple risk factors—the most common being untreated or inadequately managed mental health conditions.
> - An estimated 300–400 physicians die by suicide in the U.S. per year.
> - Physicians who took their lives were less likely to be receiving mental health treatment compared with nonphysicians who took their lives even though depression was found to be a significant risk factor at approximately the same rate in both groups.
> - The suicide rate among male physicians is 1.41 times higher than the general male population. And among female physicians, the relative risk is even more pronounced—2.27 times greater than the general female population.

_____

[1]Reprinted from American Foundation for Suicide Prevention: "Facts About Physician Depression and Suicide," in *After a Suicide: A Toolkit for Physician Residency/Fellowship Programs*. Copyright 2018, American Foundation for Suicide Prevention. Used with permission.

- Suicide is the second-leading cause of death in the 24–34 age range (Accidents are the first).
- Twenty-eight percent of residents experience a major depressive episode during training versus 7%–8% of similarly aged individuals in the U.S. general population.
- Among physicians, risk for suicide increases when mental health conditions go unaddressed, and self-medication occurs as a way to address anxiety, insomnia or other distressing symptoms. Although self-medicating, mainly with prescription medications, may reduce some symptoms, the underlying health problem is not effectively treated. This can lead to a tragic outcome.
- In one study, 23% of interns had suicidal thoughts. However, among those interns who completed four sessions of web-based cognitive behavior therapy, suicidal ideation decreased by nearly 50%.
- Drivers of burnout include workload, work inefficiency, lack of autonomy and meaning in work, and work-home conflict.
- Unaddressed mental health conditions, in the long run, are more likely to have a negative impact on a physician's professional reputation and practice than reaching out for help early.

So how much of this is relevant to Marco? First, we know that in their lifetime, approximately 15% of physicians will develop a substance use disorder and/or a mental health–related condition that could potentially impair their ability to practice medicine (Boisaubin and Levine 2001) as happened with him. Of particular importance in relation to suicide are burnout and depression, both of which will be addressed more extensively in Chapters 2 and 9, and both of which he exhibited at times. A particularly poignant perspective of burnout and depression and the effect that it can have on a physician has recently been recorded by Weinstein (2018), who described his illness and his recovery and made the important observation that "you would not be reading this today were it not for the love of my wife, my children, my mother and sister, and so many others, including the guards and doctors who 'locked me up' against my will. They kept me from crossing into the abyss" (p. 795).

Second, we know that physicians are at a higher risk for suicide than the general population. As the AFSP notes, the suicide rate for female physicians in particular is markedly elevated, with a relative risk of 2.27 compared with U.S. women in general, while that of male physicians is also above the U.S. national average, with a relative risk of 1.4 (Schernhammer and Colditz 2004). What this means is that, all other things being equal, physicians are more likely to kill themselves than nonphysician equivalent adults in the general population. This finding is hardly surprising, as physicians have the knowledge and skills to make sure that they are successful in a suicide attempt and consequently have a much higher rate of completed suicide in comparison to suicide attempts than does the general population. Interestingly, although suicide is still the second most common cause of death in residents, in a 14-year study of 381,000 U.S. residents by Yaghmour et al. (2017), fewer residents than individuals from an age- and gender-matched general population died by suicide, although temporal patterns showed higher rates of suicide earlier in residency and during the first and third quarters of the academic year. Partly as a result of these data, the Accreditation Council for Graduate Medical Education has introduced mandatory training on physician health as part of its professionalism curriculum, starting in 2017, as will be more extensively discussed in Chapter 10.

Third, we know that risk factors for suicide include major depression and other mood disorders, substance abuse, adverse life events, access to lethal means, medical illness, family history of mental illness, age (50 or older), and gender (male more common overall) (Haskins et al. 2016). Marco had several of these risk factors—namely, age, gender, alcohol abuse, depression, access to lethal means, and major stresses and life event changes. Gendel and colleagues (2017), in a retrospective case analysis of 70 physicians reporting suicidal thoughts compared with 1,572 who did not, have concluded that multiple stressors, which should not be viewed as transitory, are particularly significant as risk factors in physicians.

Although there is anecdotal evidence that those physicians who work in emergency departments or as anesthesiologists are most likely to die by suicide, compared with other medical specialties (mainly because they do have higher rates of narcotic addiction than other specialties), the numerous studies of physician suicide have not identified specific risk factors associated with any particular type of medical practice or specialist discipline.

Finally, we know that physicians rarely report depression or suicidal ideas freely, as was the case with Marco, who simply withdrew and missed appointments. These behaviors are embedded in the medical subculture, which encourages denial and self-reliance, and are at least partly learned implicitly during training, as was certainly the case here (Brimstone et al. 2007). Marco managed to cope professionally up to the final event that led to him being sent home from work, despite all his marital problems and family difficulties, and in that setting he continued his lifelong pattern of delaying or avoiding care and treatment at least partly because of the perceived stigma associated with mental illness.

Wible (2017) has recently written about this "suffering in silence," and having interviewed 200 physicians with depression, she identified why many doctors do nothing, preferring to put up with their problems rather than seek help; normalizing their own misery; and using distraction, denial, and avoidance. She found that as an alternative, self-treatment was a common option, with choices ranging from maintaining obsessive levels of exercise and reading multiple self-help books to self-prescribing or quitting medicine altogether. The consequence is that it is common for physicians to be either untreated or undertreated for depression and similar disorders, which only increases their risk of suicide.

Michael Myers (2017) has also written extensively about this issue, noting how the strengths and vulnerabilities of physicians, combined with the culture of medicine and what he called the "fight not to become a patient" that many physicians demonstrate, are core reasons why physicians remain untreated when they are depressed, and how this also increases their risk of suicide. Fortunately, he also describes how effectively depression can be treated and suicide can potentially be prevented through a combination of educating physicians and their families and revitalizing and changing the culture of medicine, as is discussed in several other chapters.

While Marco's tragic story brings up many other possible points for discussion, one more needs to be mentioned. What was the impact of his death on his family and on his carers—his wife and family, his psychiatrist, his colleagues, and his friends and community members? All were present at his funeral. All must surely have had mixed feelings of grief, loss, disbelief, frustration, anger, guilt, and self-blame. There is no easy way to cope with a situation like this, in which a loved one, a patient, a father, or a friend kills himself.

Much has been written about the impact of an individual's suicide on family and loved ones, but the suicide of a physician is without doubt rather different. No one really expects the healer to destroy himself or herself. So, while families of anyone who has died by suicide go through the well-described grief process of denial, anger, acceptance, and resolution, the frequent additional anger and feelings of hopelessness and betrayal seen with a physician suicide tend to make the grief and healing process longer and more delayed than in deaths due, for instance, to natural causes. After all, the physician patient who has died by suicide is both the victim and the perpetrator of the final fatal event. This is very different from most deaths and almost inevitably leads to ambivalent mixed feelings in loved ones, both anger at the person and loss and sadness at the outcome, as well as in many cases guilt and self-blame. A whole range of emotions is seen in family members and friends of those who have died by suicide. These range from intense guilt at not having prevented the suicide, through a sense of failure and confusion that their family member felt unloved and killed himself or herself, to distress over a range of unresolved issues, some of which might have contributed to the suicide.

A number of follow-up studies of family and friends of those who have died by suicide have demonstrated significant, and quite common, short- and long-term impacts on both their physical and mental health, as well as a greater likelihood of further suicides and suicide attempts in this group itself. One of the causes of this is the stigma that almost inevitably surrounds the death. When someone dies, the usual social responses are to offer compassion and empathy, but when the death is by suicide, the loved ones of the person who died by suicide are often treated very differently and are themselves less likely to talk about the suicide because they are concerned they will be judged and condemned. This may lead to further isolation and feelings of loss and sadness, and sometimes thereafter to maladaptive responses, such as self-medication with alcohol, overeating, and nonadherence to healthy lifestyles. All of these responses can make preexisting medical conditions like diabetes or heart disease worse and may contribute to increased depression and anxiety.

Given the impact of suicide on families and friends, what then are the effects on a clinician when his or her patient dies by suicide? For mental health workers, and psychiatrists in particular, it is important to recognize that suicide, never mind physician suicide, is best thought of as an occupational hazard, just as is, for surgeons, an unexpected death during an operation. Numerous studies have reported that at least 50% of psychiatrists will have a patient die by suicide whom they know well and are treating regularly, at least once during their career. Not surprisingly this can cause quite severe distress, especially in younger clinicians who may not have had to confront the possibility of a death of someone they know well, and care for, by suicide. Such distress can focus on treatment decisions, and whether these were right or not, and can initiate a fear of criticism from colleagues or retribution from lawsuits. Individual reactions to such deaths, not surprisingly, vary enormously. It is not uncommon for emotional reactions following a patient's death by suicide to include serious self-doubt about a career choice, trauma-related symptoms and reactions, and overly cautious future clinical behavior, leading to excessive numbers of patients being hospitalized and generally defensive clinical practice approaches. Conversely, some physicians accept the event as an almost predictable outcome in a few patients along the lines of observers of war who talk about civilian casualties occurring during firefights as predictable, regrettable, but unavoidable "collateral damage."

Whatever the physician's emotional response, there are some practical tasks that need to be attended to by physicians following a patient suicide. These include notifying their malpractice insurer and reviewing the events leading up to the suicide, commonly thought of as a "psychological autopsy" or a "sentinel event" or "risk management" review. These processes are frequently laid out in hospital policy manuals and are used for any sort of unexpected death or major adverse clinical event. They are best performed with some supportive colleagues and in a manner that is ideally primarily educational rather than investigatory so as not to prematurely provide either blame or reassurance that the death was somehow inevitable. Sometimes such reviews are not possible, especially in private practice, where a practitioner may be relatively isolated from other colleagues, and in these instances meeting with a mentor or colleague to talk through the event is sensible.

In the case described in this chapter, one of the tasks involved following up with the family of the patient, bearing in mind any important confidentiality and privacy issues, and even going to the funeral. This is not something that all physicians feel comfortable doing; it is a matter of personal choice and dependent on the clinician's prior relationship with the patient's family and the situation. Some physicians continue to see spouses or other family relations of their patients who have died by suicide as patients or continue to provide reassurance and empathic support to community members of a deceased patient. Such relationships may last for several years and be helpful and therapeutic for the family members and sometimes, vicariously, for the physician.

References

American Foundation for Suicide Prevention: Facts about physician depression and suicide, in After a Suicide: A Toolkit for Physician Residency/Fellowship Programs. 2018. Available at: https://afsp.org/our-work/education/physician-medical-student-depression-suicide-prevention/#section1. Accessed January 16, 2018.

American Medical Association: STEPS forward. Preventing physician distress and suicide. 2018. Available at: https://www.stepsforward.org/modules/preventing-physician-suicide. Accessed January 16, 2018.

Boisaubin EV, Levine RE: Identifying and assisting the impaired physician. Am J Med Sci 322(1):31–36, 2001

Brooks E: Preventing physician distress and suicide. American Medical Association, Steps Forward series, 2018. Available at: https://www.stepsforward.org/modules/preventing-physician-suicide. Accessed January 16, 2018.

Brimstone R, Thistlethwaite JE, Quirk F: Behaviour of medical students in seeking mental and physical health care: exploration and comparison with psychology students. Med Educ 41(1):74–83, 2007 17209895

Center C, Davis M, Detre T, et al: Confronting depression and suicide in physicians: a consensus statement. JAMA 289(23):3161–3166, 2003 12813122

Gendel MH, Early SR, et al: When doctors struggle: current stressors and evaluation recommendations for physicians contemplating suicide. Arch Suicide Res Oct 9, 2017 [Epub ahead of print] 28990863

Haskins J, Carson JG, Chang CH, et al: The suicide prevention, depression awareness, and clinical engagement program for faculty and residents at the University of California, Davis Health System. Acad Psychiatry 40(1):23–29, 2016 26063680

Myers M: Why Physicians Die by Suicide: Lessons Learned From Their Families and Others Who Cared. San Bernadino, CA, 2017

Rose JS, Campbell MD, Yellowlees P, et al: Family medicine physicians with substance use disorder: a 5-year outcome study. J Addict Med 11(2):93–97, 2017 28067757

Schernhammer ES, Colditz GA: Suicide rates among physicians: a quantitative and gender assessment (meta-analysis). Am J Psychiatry 161(12):2295–2302, 2004 15569903

Weinstein MS. Out of the straitjacket. N Engl J Med 378:793–795, 2018

Wible PL: Doctors and depression: suffering in silence. May 11, 2017. Available at: http://www.medscape.com/viewarticle/879379. Accessed January 16, 2018.

Yaghmour NA, Brigham TP, Richter T, et al: Causes of death of residents in ACGME-accredited programs 2000 through 2014: implications for the learning environment. Acad Med 92(7):976–983, 2017 28514230

Trapped at Work

DR. TINA GARLAND seemed anxious and hesitated as I called her name in the waiting area. She stood out in the crowded room with her conservative gray suit, black pumps, and white silk scarf tied closely around her neck. Her hair was pulled back away from her face by a headband. She had obviously tried to camouflage the deep dark circles around her eyes with heavy makeup. The immediate impression was of someone trying desperately to hide exhaustion. She followed me down the corridor to my office and sat down on the edge of the chair. "Good morning, Dr. Garland," I said. "It's good to meet you. I understand you have been having some difficulty at your work. What can I do for you?"

"I don't know why I am here. I don't think you will be able to help, but things have been going badly at work. It's getting harder each day to get dressed and make it into work. I'm so tired all the time. I just can't keep going like I am. My nurse who has been with me for many years took me aside and gave me your details—she said I needed to come and see you. She told me that you had a lot of physicians for patients and that she was going to quit my practice if I didn't at least try to get some help. I know she's right. I'm not myself anymore."

"How about you tell me a little more about yourself? I understand you are a pediatrician and you work in the large downtown clinic."

"'Working' is an understatement—I feel like I live there. Like I'm trapped. Maybe I will move my bed permanently into my office," she continued in an exasperated manner.

"After all, my children wouldn't miss me—they never see me now. I spend so much time at home on the computer in the evenings and weekends catching up with notes that my youngest daughter asked me the other day if I was a computer person and was that my job. You know the old saying "Out of the mouths of babes"—well, I think she was right. That's all I seem to do nowadays—sit and type. Spending rewarding time with patients is a thing of the past. I have to take less time with my patients—spending time with my patients is what I really like to do—because I need more time for the health record work. My work just doesn't seem meaningful anymore and it's ruining my family life."

She continued: "You know what makes me most angry? It's all the administrative work that takes away from patient care. I don't get any time to do the little extra things that my patients, and my own kids, used to love me for. I miss getting my kids to draw and color or playing board games with them. I was teaching them chess, but it's been so long I'm not sure I know how to play anymore. I don't have time to call parents back to check on things, like I used to do. Instead, I spend ages doing insurance authorizations and excessive documentation, and everyone wants a piece of me. I have a full day of patients—one every 15 minutes. They just keep on coming in an unending line that never stops. I feel totally out of control. I cannot keep up with them. God forbid one has a crisis and I have to spend more than the allocated 15 minutes. The entire day is ruined. I never get a lunch-break, and I always finish late."

She resumed her continuous monologue as if a dam had begun to break and she had to let all of her irritation flow out. "It's not their fault, but I can feel myself trying to rush them and their moms out of the room, hoping they don't have any extra problems that will take up more time. I feel I have lost the human side of medicine and am beginning to think of my patients as objects that I have to service and get out of my clinic so I can finish. It feels all wrong, and I hate it. I went into medicine to spend time with people, and I used to so love being a pediatrician and all the time I spent with families. I used to get lots of thank-you notes, but that hasn't happened in a while. Now I have to write repetitive notes in the EMR [electronic medical record] that take so long just to make sure we get paid for my services. Most of what I have to write is not really about good patient care— it's just to satisfy all the bean counters in the system. It all makes me feel totally frustrated and constantly irritated. No wonder I get annoyed with my staff and colleagues. I guess it's not surprising that my nurse sent me off to see a psychiatrist. Don't you think that it's a bit ironic that that is a sign that she cares for me?"

Tina's emotional dam burst then and there. She spoke relentlessly about a series of situations that were occurring at her work, and how she felt frustrated, angry, and helpless at being unable to deliver the sort of care she felt her patients needed and that she had been used to providing in previous jobs. It was fascinating listening to Tina as she angrily described in herself a classic case of burnout. She continued talking and illustrated in detail the three main areas of symptoms that typically are considered to be signs of burnout: exhaustion, emotional distancing from her work, and reduced performance at work and home. In her case this meant being physically tired and lacking sleep, working on her computer to do notes at all hours of the day and night, resenting her patients and their families for being the cause of her workload, and feeling anger at her husband for not helping with their own children more.

I sat back and listened sympathetically, as this was something that I had seen and heard so frequently before in many physicians whom I had helped. Finally, she took a deep breath and stopped herself.

"Are there any other issues that are worrying you?" I asked.

This previously well put together and sophisticated physician completely broke down in front of me and burst into floods of tears.

"Where would you like me to start? My life is a mess. My marriage is a disaster. My children never see me. I can't cope anymore. The world seems so dark, so empty. Sometimes I just wish I could go to sleep and never wake up. Not really. I have no actual plan to kill myself. I couldn't do that to my children. They don't deserve that. At times I do find myself thinking of death as being a possible way out. I just cannot believe I've gotten to this point. I put such a good face on for everyone, and inside I'm constantly aching. Sometimes I go into my bedroom when I'm alone and just cry myself to sleep. Sometimes I wish I could just go to sleep and not wake up—that would be such a relief."

I sat and listened and waited for her to get it all out.

"How much time have you got?" Tina asked. "I have so many problems and so little hope."

"Tell me the big issues that you have not mentioned so far. Give me a bit of an understanding of some of the reasons for your distress. You mentioned that your marriage is a disaster."

"It is. Jim is basically a good man. I still love him. But I know he cheated on me once in the past, 5 years ago, and we kept together with a lot of marriage counseling. Now I think he might be cheating again. He has disappeared a few times and has had weak excuses for where he was. He has suddenly started going to the gym more and is looking after himself better. He bought some new clothes recently. He never used to care about what he wore. I've always had to drag him to shop for clothes, but lately he doesn't even want me to go with him. I'm sure it's partly my fault that we have drifted apart. We haven't had sex for over a year—I just don't feel like it and don't want him physically near me. So we're living like roommates—being polite to each other, despite my suspicions, and making sure the children are looked after and making sure our friends think we are solid as a couple. But we aren't. We're distant. It feels like a sort of truce that we're both afraid to break because if we do, something worse may happen. And I just don't know what to do about it. So we're going to have to talk about that. I need your advice as this cannot go on."

I explored further. "Tell me about your children and how you're getting on with them by yourself and as a couple."

"You know, kids are amazing. That is one of the reasons I went into pediatrics after medical school. They're so resilient. I wish they could teach us some of their skills. Robbie is 10, and all he's interested in is soccer. Is there such a thing as a soccer addict? As long as there is a ball and a game to talk about, he's fine. My neighbor's son is on the same soccer team, so she's getting my son to practice and to the games. I know he gets upset with me—with how irritable I am—and he sometimes comes and sits next to me and puts his arm around me. How is it that my 10-year-old is reverse-caring for me and that he's such a comfort? Anyway I think he is fine and doing well at school and has lots of friends. Ann is 7, and I don't think she really understands how upset I am, although she has recently started wetting her bed after a year of being dry. I'm worried that I'm the cause of that—and of course having to get up at night to change her bed doesn't help my sleep. I wish Jim would help more, but he just seems disinterested and unaware. I do worry about her, and I see so much of myself in her. She has always been a worrier, just like me, and I know she will be affected by our situation."

"Let's circle back to them later. What about your physical health? I saw in your notes that you had breast cancer…"

"Yes. That was 3 years ago. I'm sure that's one of the causes of our marriage situation. Jim got really frightened and physically avoided me while I was going through reconstruction surgery. I felt he was grossed out by my bald head. He didn't say so, but I knew he was. I never let Jim see my chest after surgery mainly because I was sure it was too much for him. The reconstruction has come out really well, but we don't ever talk about the surgery or the way I am now. It's another thing we've just never worked through as a couple. And I can't help blaming myself for that. I know he must find me unattractive, but I've always really done my best to look good for him. At least I'm cancer-free physically, but I'm so screwed up emotionally. I know I need help. I just can't survive the way things are now. Something has to change."

By the end of this first session—one full of trauma for Tina—we had agreed on a plan of action. I was seriously concerned about her safety, but she was prepared to contract with me not to harm herself and to visit regularly for therapy. She agreed to start antidepressants for her depressive illness, and I educated her about these. She also agreed to do some reading about burnout and depression. I gave her a number of Web sites and URLs to look at on these topics. She committed to talking to her clinic medical director to see if her workload could be reduced somewhat, although she made it clear that she was not going to take any sick leave, which I had suggested. Then we agreed to start to meet on a regular basis, initially weekly, so that I could get to know her better and she could work with me on her therapy, which was going to be extensive.

The following week Tina returned late one afternoon. This time she was angry and distressed. "I have just had the most horrendous day at work. I cannot believe what has happened to me. I've read all those articles you gave me on burnout, and they fit me perfectly. How could I possibly have gotten to be like this? I've just been trying to do my best. The whole health system has been fighting against me. Even after a day like this I still have notes to write on 10 patients and a full EMR inbox with messages from patients and questions or directives from colleagues and administrators. I have to go back to work after this session and will be there for another couple of hours at least. Let me give you an example of what happened this morning—of why my whole day was destroyed."

I listened as she went into great detail about what had happened to her. At one point she began pacing around the room almost yelling about how her workload was so extreme that she just could not keep up with it all. She described her staff as unsupportive and some patients as "too needy." She finally collapsed in her chair and just sobbed. At least she had a safe place to explode, to get her frustration off her chest. I hoped this could allow her to ventilate in front of me and avoid such a scene for her family. I felt that Tina needed this safe place so she could talk freely and not be judged. "I thought today was going to be a good day at last, after a bad couple of weeks. I checked yesterday evening and I had a full day of patients booked today, but I know them all and none worried me. So I was expecting a fairly routine clinic and hoping I would be able to maybe even catch up on a few of my backlogged notes. Well, stupid me. I arrived at work to find that my clinic had been completely rearranged. One of the other doctors was off sick and all of his patients had been redistributed with no notice, and guess who had been given more than her fair share? Why do they think I can always just do everything? The first patient's family I had to see were well-known "challenges"—both parents drug addicts and constantly trying to have their children, who do not have ADHD [attention-deficit/hyperactivity disorder], put on stimulants. Who knows, maybe they wanted the drugs for themselves. They've complained about me in the past when I haven't given them the drugs they wanted, but the clinic administration has refused to fire them as patients despite several of us mere doctors being verbally attacked and abused by them. Well, I had to deal with them, and the only way to do that was to take double the time of a normal appointment. So by the time I even got to my first patient, I was half an hour behind, and of course my own patients were now complaining at being kept waiting. The first mother had especially booked the first appointment of the day to be able to get elsewhere rapidly. At the same time my EMR inbox had filled up and I could see there were not just the usual patient queries but also several urgent "prior authorizations" from insurers. I cannot stand those—they are just a way for the payers to get out of paying for services, and they can take ages to do. So I'm already upset and frustrated, but I get my patient into my room and am trying to pay attention to her when my door opens and a medical student walks in. Can you believe it? Today of all days."

Tina paused to take a deep breath and calm herself before continuing: "Now normally I like having students, but not today without any warning. I later found out it wasn't their fault, as this was planned some time ago, but I knew nothing about them coming in today to shadow me, and while having a student is good, it does take more time since you have to explain and teach more to both them and the patients. Not a good day for it today, but I had no choice because I was the only general pediatrician in the clinic at that time, and that was the rotation they were doing. Anyway, I soldier on, with every patient being late, and not even attempting to keep up with my EMR notes, knowing they would be done in the evening, and it was simply one of those days. Everything that could go wrong went wrong. Patients' results were not available. Everyone was being seen late and fed up with waiting. I wrote a couple of prescriptions incorrectly—you know the usual constantly changing rules for controlled substances—and had pharmacies phoning me urgently to correct them. Extra patients inserted by the clinic staff as a result of my sick colleague—it makes the front desk staff look good in the patients' eyes when they accommodate patients, but they don't have to actually see the extra people themselves and with minimal or no time available. And on top of that, one of my patients had some really serious medical problems, and I had to counsel her and her family, all of whom were very upset, while all I wanted to do was get out of the room and escape. I really couldn't feel as empathic with them as I would have liked, which is not like me, and I just wanted to get the session over. It almost felt like each of my patients ended up just being a number on a list that I was struggling to get through."

She sighed and reflected. "The day from hell. Where I felt, and was, completely out of control all day. Everyone wanting bits of me. And always immediately. No time for anything for myself, and it just feels like a crowd that you have to fight your way through, except the crowd keeps getting larger and more aggressive, and you feel like you are about to get pushed under. The only good thing that happened all day was my nurse taking me aside and forcing me to sit down and have a cup of coffee she had made for me, and quietly checking that I had come to see you. I think she was the only person who thought of me in a positive way all day. Everyone else just wanted to control what I did and use parts of me, and that is how I felt all day—used and controlled. The sad part about this is that while today was exceptionally bad, I've been feeling like this almost all days for ages now. So it's not unusual for me."

Tina continued to see me on a weekly basis and, with a combination of antidepressants, supportive therapy, and suggestions as to how she could modify her lifestyle and work arrangements, seemed to gradually start to improve.

Suddenly 6 weeks later she called me in tears: "I just can't cope any longer. I need to see you immediately. It all seems so hopeless. I can't deal with it anymore. I just want it all to end."

I met with her urgently a few hours later: "I know you're doing your best to help me," Tina said, "but there's really no point. My marriage with Jim is over. He has moved out and said he is going to fight me to keep the kids. He says I'm a pathetic mother. That I spend more time at work than home and that when I'm home I ignore them all anyway. The children seem to go to Jim and don't even ask me for permission to go places anymore. I know he's exaggerating, but there's some truth in it, and maybe they would be better off without me. I'm really not feeling much better than when I first saw you. I tried to put on a brave face and didn't want to disappoint you, so I've been telling you I was feeling better on the meds, but I'm really not. I stopped taking the meds after 1 week and just lied to you about that. I am not managing my work and am constantly afraid of making a serious mistake—today I completely forgot to order some important labs on a new child I saw because I just felt under too much pressure to finish the consultation rapidly and see my other patients. I can't sleep, and I'm constantly worrying about my work and going over what I've done to make sure I haven't made any mistakes. I'm just not coping. What can I do? Please help me."

This was serious, and I decided to focus on Dr. Garland's safety initially: "So, Tina, tell me about what you mean when you say you want to 'end it all.'"

"Well, I have a large collection of pills at home that have built up over time. I look at them in the medicine cabinet in my bathroom at home every evening and know that if I took them all they would be enough. I've thought about just quietly taking them at night so that I would be dead by morning, but I can't stand the thought of my children finding me dead, so I've looked up some hotels not too far outside of town where I could get away by myself. Alternatively, I could get the children to stay at my sister's for the weekend and then do it while they are away—at least they wouldn't find me and have that awful memory to live with."

She looked at me in desperation. "The other alternative would be just to self-inject myself—I could easily get some potassium vials from work and combine them with a sedative and just get it over with quickly. But I don't want to be found out doing this, and I worry that my children might come in unexpectedly at home. I've even thought of taking a bath and cutting my radial arteries and slowly bleeding out. I never used to think that one of the advantages of being a doctor is that we would know how to kill ourselves properly, but it's true. I can think of lots of ways. I just seem to be obsessed with these thoughts, and although part of me doesn't want to do anything like this, it's just scary. Please help me. I just don't trust myself anymore. These thoughts keep coming into my mind and I'm so torn. I know I don't want to die most of the time, but sometimes those feelings are overwhelming and it seems like it might be better for everyone if I did finally kill myself. Just get it all over. It's so painful going through this day after day."

Three months later I was sitting with Tina during one of our weekly sessions reviewing how she was getting on. She was looking better and was dressed casually in a tracksuit, with her hair in a ponytail and a little makeup. She no longer looked exhausted and was able to smile and interact much more warmly with me than she had in the past. She knew that I had nearly legally certified her and hospitalized her against her will for her own safety, but that instead of this, she had agreed to take a month off work and have her parents come and stay with her to help look after the children and herself. She agreed to me talking to her parents, but not her husband, to emphasize the gravity of the situation, and to restart her medication. She had then gone back to work on a half-time basis only, as part of a carefully planned rehab program involving a lot of lifestyle changes, including the addition of regular exercise and yoga. Rather to my surprise, and despite her concern about the stigma of seeing a psychiatrist, she also allowed me to discuss possible adaptations to her workload with her clinic medical director so that she could reduce the workplace stresses that were one of the causes of burnout that had clearly been a precipitant, among others, of her severe depressive illness.

"What's happening with you and Jim?" I asked.

"I'm just not sure. We do seem to be getting on somewhat better and even had a date night last week when we went out to see a movie together. We went for dessert and coffee afterwards and started to really talk for the first time in years."

I encouraged her to continue.

She resumed, hesitantly at first: "I finally had the nerve to confront him with my fears that he might have been cheating again, and he absolutely denied it. He responded very differently from the last time when I had found out about his cheating. Then he had become angry and defensive and had immediately denied everything. This time he listened to me and said he had left because he just couldn't stand being in the same house as me and that I had been constantly critical, suspicious, and angry with him. And with the children. He could see that I had changed and was not myself, but he had gotten to the end of his rope and couldn't think of anything to do to help me. He said he had even wondered if I had had some sort of recurrence of my breast cancer that was affecting me psychologically, but he was afraid to bring this up as he thought I would bite his head off. It seems that he got on the Internet and looked up all the psychological aftereffects and impacts of breast cancer and read about how women commonly get depression afterwards. He said he finally thought it might actually be better if we were apart and I had more space to sort myself out with your help, but as you know he only left for a few weeks before returning, thank goodness. I think it was good that my mom moved in for a while because that gave us all a bit of space and she was able to focus on looking after the children while I took a break to try and get myself together. I'm not sure I completely believe him and his denials about not cheating, but at least it's out in the open now and is something we can discuss and hopefully work through. Certainly, I feel less actively suspicious of him, and he hasn't been doing anything odd or unusual recently. He actually asked me if I would go with him to marriage counseling, which is a first and which shows motivation on his part, I guess. So we would like your advice about who might be helpful for us, please."

"That's good, Tina. I'm pleased. I'll certainly give you a list of possible therapists you can contact. It's best that you see someone independent who neither of you has seen before so that neither of you feels disadvantaged as you go through marital counseling. Let's shift tracks. Tell me how you're finding work now that you've been back part-time for a few weeks."

Tina brightened up at this and responded positively. "Well, that has actually been a pleasant surprise. You know, one of the good things to come out of this whole episode is that I've begun to understand how much I'm valued at work, although it strikes me as odd that we never get told that. I just couldn't see it before. Now that I look back I can see that I was completely burned out for months before I ever came to see you. My nurse took me aside the other day and told me how nice it is to have "the old me" back again. She said she was really pleased, and we ended up having a really nice friendly hug right in the middle of the clinic! I am still having dreadful trouble keeping up with the EMR though, and as you know, I'm trying to limit the number of hours I spend catching up on my patient notes so that I spend a maximum of an hour extra per day. Did I tell you that my medical director arranged for one of the tech support people to come and sit in with me for a couple of days of clinic to observe how I work and to teach me how to use the EMR more efficiently? Why didn't that happen years ago? It made me think about how I was trained to use the EMR—just one session of 2 hours about 7 years ago when I started work. I had no idea there were so many shortcuts, and now that I'm able to dictate my notes using the automated systems, I'm so much quicker. I know I have a long way to go to be able to complete my notes fully within the clinic time, but I can at least see some hope at the end of the tunnel. And I plan on keeping up to date with whatever changes they put in the EMR and going to all the trainings I can to stay that way."

I decided to explore her burnout and her previously rather cynical views toward her patients further: "How are you finding your interactions with your patients?"

"You know, those are going so much better. Most of my consultations seem more meaningful to me, and I'm getting more pleasure from them. And my patients are picking that up from me, especially the younger children, who are more playful and amusing. It is just like the old days a few years ago. I'm starting to find more joy in practicing medicine. After all, that's why I wanted to become a doctor in the first place. I just feel like a very different person, with a changed attitude and approach. I know I have to go back to full-time work soon, and that will probably be hard in some respects, but if Jim and I can get our marriage sorted out, then I hope we'll take more holidays. Eventually, if his career takes off more, I may even be able to cut my hours back a bit and have more time for myself and my family."

"That all sounds very positive, Tina. I just want to check that you no longer have suicidal ideas and that you're feeling completely safe, and not just telling me what you think I want to hear. Remember how you did that before." I had learned to double-check everything with Tina because of her tendency to want to impress me and deny the severity of her illness. She was like a true frontline soldier who would always press on whatever the stress and pressure until she got to her breaking point.

"I understand why you ask that. Don't worry. I really am no longer suicidal. I'm positive about the future now and will continue to see you, take my meds, and participate in therapy. But I just cannot believe how close I got to killing myself. I was in a very dark place. I felt physically exhausted and hopeless, with no future and no support, so suicide actually seemed to be a logical way out of my gloom. And as you know I got rather obsessed about it. I don't know if I would have done it or not. But I do know that I thought about it a great deal and worked out a number of ways of killing myself that would not have been too painful or distressing, but that would have been effective. I didn't want any more pain than I already had with my depression, so the trick for me at the time was to work out a painless way of killing myself—a bit like just falling asleep and never waking up. I didn't tell you about it, but at one stage I even thought of driving full speed into a tree, but I dismissed shooting or hanging myself since those would have been just too painful for me and would have disfigured my body so much that it would have been distressing for my family to see if they found me. When I look back, it's just amazing how much detail you can think about a terrible topic like this. That all seems a long time ago. I'm not in that negative space anymore."

As Dr. Garland continued to get better and recovered from her depression with a combination of medications, improvements in her work-life balance, marital therapy, and her own therapy with me, I started to see her less frequently, and a year after her initial referral I was just seeing her monthly as she continued to progress in a positive direction. I was now meeting with a woman who was much more confident; who looked physically stronger, having put on a little weight, but who no longer had dark circles under her eyes; and who tended to lead most of the sessions we had by discussing topics of immediate importance to herself. I decided to try to make her reflect more deeply on her recent experience and asked her to review what she thought had changed for and around her during the course of the past year and how she felt this had affected her.

She considered my question carefully before answering. "Well, we talked a lot about control and the importance of meaning in all aspects of my life. They are the two big issues that I think have changed, and which make me much more confident about going forward."

She paused, sat up a bit straighter, and looked out of the window at the beautiful spring day before continuing. "I really think that I'm much more settled and comfortable with Jim. We have a much better relationship and are both working hard on being loving and respectful to each other. We have stopped being roommates and are now honest about our feelings. We have worked through some of the misconceptions we had about each other when I dealt with cancer and my mastectomies. It turns out Jim felt I was pushing him out, and looking back I probably was. I was so angry and afraid and I wouldn't talk with him. I didn't give him a chance to help me through that horrible year. We've been getting away for long weekends by ourselves, which has brought us close again and has really helped our sex life. I know that we still occasionally have a flare of tempers, but even that is better than just flat politeness. So I think we're both much more confident about our long-term future, and I, in particular, have managed to make more time for both him and the kids, so as a family we're way different. We're still not there yet, and I think we'll continue going to the marriage therapist for a while yet, but at least we are both now motivated to change and are giving ourselves a chance. You know, it's interesting now that I think about it that I focused on that element of my life first. In the past I would have jumped straight in to talk about work."

"Good point," I said. "So what about your work?"

"Well, that has changed quite dramatically, and more than I've perhaps really told you in the past. Gerard, the clinic medical director, really took my illness to heart and saw it as a sign he had to make dramatic changes so that no one else would suffer like I had. He has been quite funny about it and regularly checks on me, describing me as his clinic thermometer! If I'm feeling OK, the temperature of the clinic is probably OK! But seriously, there have been some systemic changes, and all the clinical staff, doctors, and patients are feeling much better, and I think we are delivering better care. Gerard organized a number of internal symposia on burnout, and we all read about it and what works best to prevent it and have been following up with monthly meetings to make changes and monitor how the clinic is working and how we are all feeling. I really feel I'm being listened to now. I suggested changing our rooming process so that the assistants did more of the busywork on the EMR, and that has made a huge difference and saves me at least 2 minutes of documentation per patient, which really adds up. And while not all my ideas get taken up, some certainly do. It's just so good to know that I and the other doctors and nurses are being listened to. It makes us feel more in control and better respected."

I responded, "That's excellent. Can you give me some other concrete examples?"

"Sure. Yesterday Gerard announced that he wants us to create a strategic plan for the clinic and asked us all to be involved. Amazingly we've been given more administrative support, and we're getting some regular admin time each week to work on the strategic plan. So hopefully we'll develop some objectives and aims that will be accepted, and that will mean that we have had a real impact on the future direction of the clinic, and the type of care we provide, rather than just being rote providers, which is how I certainly used to see myself. We are getting more involved in other ways. We have a policy on what happens with last-minute cancellations due to sickness that we have all developed together, and of course we're getting more and regular training on our nemesis, the EMR, so that we've become more efficient and don't need to work on notes on nights and weekends. So it's all very positive, and we have to keep it up, but the good news is that all of us MDs at the clinic are planning on staying on now, whereas before, several doctors were threatening to leave. Things are going better for everyone now."

Commentary

Unfortunately, Dr. Garland's story of burnout and depression is very common, but so is her good outcome, a reflection of the many changes she made in her home and work life, her seeking and adhering to treatment, and, perhaps most importantly, her own internal strength and resilience. She had a complicated situation made worse by breast cancer, and she tried to struggle through by herself initially without getting the sort of help and counseling she would certainly have advised for one of her patients.

Much is written about burnout, but it's still a poorly understood concept or disorder. Burnout is not classified as a formal psychiatric disorder, although it may well be someday. In short, it's generally believed to be a syndrome or a group of symptoms and beliefs that are work related and that cause the individual, be he or she a doctor, nurse, engineer, lawyer, or pilot, substantial distress and disillusionment with his or her work. Maslach and Jackson (1981) wrote about it in their seminal paper describing the Maslach Burnout Inventory, still the most highly regarded measure of burnout available, when they called burnout "a syndrome of emotional exhaustion and cynicism that occurs frequently among individuals who do 'people-work' of some kind. A key aspect of the burnout syndrome is increased feelings of emotional exhaustion. As their emotional resources are depleted, workers feel they are no longer able to give of themselves at a psychological level" (p. 99). In this original research, more than 1,000 adults in a variety of health and service occupations (police, counselors, social workers, psychiatrists, psychologists, attorneys, physicians, nurses, agency administrators, teachers, and probation officers) were tested, and three subscales indicating burnout emerged from a massive amount of data:

1. Emotional exhaustion (an individual stress response)
2. Cynicism (depersonalization and a negative reaction to work)
3. Professional inefficacy (a negative evaluation of self and of personal accomplishments)

Since then, literally thousands of articles have appeared in the literature. When the search term "burnout" is entered into PubMed, the premier peer-reviewed literature search engine, 12,520 articles appear, with recent articles focusing on burnout in combat veterans, nurses, civil servants, teachers, and parents. Quite a demonstration of the breadth of interest in this syndrome.

In the medical literature the full syndrome of burnout is now more specifically defined as a syndrome comprising all three of the following, although most people affected have varying components of these sets of symptoms at any one time:

- *Emotional depletion*—the individual feels emotionally depleted, tired of going to work, and frustrated and finds it hard to deal with other people in the workplace.
- *Detachment and cynicism*—the person is less empathic with patients and feels detached from his or her work, seeing and treating patients as objects or diagnoses, rather than humans, that are primarily sources of frustration to be dealt with in whatever way is possible.
- *Low personal achievement*—the individual experiences work as unrewarding and feels as if it is not meaningful (which is why many people go into human service occupations) and as if he or she is just going through the motions.

There have been many large-scale surveys of physicians over the years, and almost all of these have indicated that physicians have higher rates of burnout, typically around 30%–40%, than other professionals. In a nationwide survey of 35,922 U.S. physicians, with 6,880 respondents, Shanafelt and his colleagues (2015) at the Mayo Clinic reported that in 2011, 45% of all physicians surveyed endorsed at least one symptom set of burnout, and in 2015 the level was 54%, a rate that, as the authors noted, was higher than for the U.S. workforce generally. A similar 2017 lifestyle survey of more than 14,000 physicians by Medscape (2017) also reported burnout rates trending upward, with the disciplines of emergency medicine, obstetrics-gynecology, and family/internal medicine having the highest rates of self-reported burnout (55%–59%), while psychiatry, allergy, ophthalmology, and pathology had the lowest, but still with rates of 42%–43%. Interestingly, a recent survey of medical students by Dyrbye et al. (2014) showed that at entry to medical school, students have lower rates of burnout than equivalent populations, but that during years 1–4 of medical school they develop higher rates compared with age-matched men and women and also report more self-rated depression and worse quality of life. This is good evidence of the impact of culture in the workplace on physicians, and a 2017 Physician Lifestyle report from Medscape concluded that burnout rates for physicians continue to trend upward, with an average of 51% reporting symptoms (Medscape 2017). In this survey, physicians from emergency medicine (59%), obstetrics-gynecology (56%) and family/internal medicine (55%) reported the highest rates, while physicians from psychiatry (42%) and allergy, ophthalmology, and pathology (43%) reported the lowest. This report indicated that too many bureaucratic tasks, too many hours at work, feeling like a cog in a wheel, and the increasing computerization of practice (e.g., EMR) were rated as the main causes by the respondents, with female doctors reporting more burnout (55%) than males (45%) and being less happy overall.

In this case Tina had a full hand of symptoms of burnout that had developed over time, and she demonstrated the personal impact of the syndrome with her suffering and distress, the potential for medical errors, and the reduced satisfaction of her patients and other staff, as well as her own reduced enjoyment of her work. She had even been thinking of changing her job, and ultimately she took quite a lot of time off work—actions that are seen commonly in high-burnout environments, where employee absenteeism and turnover rates frequently mirror the rates of burnout. Tina was somewhat unusual, however, in that she developed a severe depressive illness, with the burnout being one of the stressors leading to this, along with her marital and physical problems, and likely some genetic and personality-related predisposition. Shanafelt and Noseworthy (2017) have described the interactions and repercussions of burnout at both personal and professional levels. These include, at a personal level, broken relationships, alcohol and substance use, depression, and suicide and, at a professional level, decreased quality of care, with increased medical errors, decreased patient satisfaction, reduced professional productivity and effort, and finally increased physician turnover.

So what is the overlap between burnout and more severe psychiatric disorders such as depression, alcohol and substance use, anxiety, and post-traumatic stress? The honest answer is that we're not currently sure, and this is an area where a lot more research is needed. In the case of Tina, there was substantial overlap between her burnout, on the one hand, and relationship problems and depression, on the other, and treating the latter involved managing the former, which she did well. It is likely that burnout is, in people who are biologically or psychologically vulnerable to developing depression, a stressor, just like many other psychosocial stressors, and this would explain why only a relatively small number of physicians end up, as Tina did, developing a severe depressive disorder following an episode of burnout. Indeed, burnout itself tends in most people to be self-limiting; in other words, the symptoms remit over time most likely because individuals' behavior has changed, or there have been alterations in their work environment that make them feel more valued and in control, just as was seen with Tina and her colleagues.

What is becoming clear is the importance and effectiveness of strategies to both prevent and reduce rates of burnout in physicians. A number of recent publications have reviewed such strategies, and the accumulated evidence for a number of solutions is strong. In an excellent systematic review of physician burnout and well-being, Rothenberger (2017) concluded:

> All U.S. medical students, physicians in training, and practicing physicians are at significant risk of burnout. Its prevalence now exceeds 50%. Burnout is the unintended net result of multiple, highly disruptive changes in society at large, the medical profession, and the healthcare system. Both individual and organizational strategies have been only partially successful in mitigating burnout and in developing resiliency and well-being among physicians. Two highly effective strategies are aligning personal and organizational values and enabling physicians to devote 20% of their work activities to the part of their medical practice that is especially meaningful to them. More research is needed. (p. 567)

In a similarly influential review, focused primarily on institutional change strategies, Shanafelt and Noseworthy (2017) concluded:

> Physician burnout has been shown to influence quality of care, patient safety, physician turnover, and patient satisfaction. Although burnout is a system issue, most institutions operate under the erroneous framework

that burnout and professional satisfaction are solely the responsibility of the individual physician. Engagement is the positive antithesis of burnout and is characterized by vigor, dedication, and absorption in work. There is a strong business case for organizations to invest in efforts to reduce physician burnout and promote engagement....Our experience demonstrates that deliberate, sustained, and comprehensive efforts by the organization to reduce burnout and promote engagement can make a difference. Many effective interventions are relatively inexpensive, and small investments can have a large impact. Leadership and sustained attention from the highest level of the organization are the keys to making progress. (p. 129)

Shanafelt and Noseworthy (2017) defined nine organizational strategies that support the processes of institutional, cultural, and individual change:

1. Acknowledge and assess the problem.
2. Harness the power of leadership.
3. Develop and implement targeted interventions.
4. Cultivate community at work.
5. Use rewards and incentives wisely.
6. Align values and strengthen culture.
7. Promote flexibility and work-life integration.
8. Provide resources to promote resilience and self-care.
9. Facilitate and fund organizational science.

These are all good strategies to create change, and are not dissimilar to those proposed in the two excellent online modules produced by the American Medical Association (AMA) (2018b, 2018c) on the prevention of burnout in both residents and physicians, which identify systems-level and individual interventions to prevent burnout. In its excellent online "STEPS Forward" series, the AMA (2018a) has set a goal to achieve a quadruple aim in healthcare, instead of the well-known national triple aim ("better care, better outcomes, and lower costs"), by adding in a fourth aim of "clinician wellness," which is focused on creating a joyful practice environment and a more engaged and satisfied medical workforce. This series quotes the three domains of the Stanford Wellness Framework (Stanford Medicine 2017), as well as a series of practical ways to implement the goals of the domains. The Stanford domains comprise the following:

1. A *culture of wellness*, through the creation of a work environments with a set of normative values, attitudes, and behaviors that promote self-care, personal and professional growth, and compassion for colleagues, patients, and self

2. *Efficiency of practice*, which is determined by dividing value-added clinical work accomplished by time and energy spent
3. *Personal resilience*, with a set of individual skills, behaviors, and attitudes that contribute to personal physical, emotional, and social well-being

Many of the symptoms and signs of burnout occur in environments where change is occurring already, with some describing a moral imperative for academic medical centers to address physician health (Blue Ridge Academic Health Group 2017–18). Not surprisingly, the literature in this area focuses strongly on change management and how change affects physicians in their workplaces (Bohman et al. 2017). The AMA (2018b) has identified nine steps to help clinicians through such organizational changes:

1. Engage senior leadership.
2. Track the business case for well-being.
3. Resource a wellness infrastructure.
4. Measure burnout and the predictors of burnout longitudinally.
5. Strengthen local leadership.
6. Develop interventions and evaluate their impact.
7. Improve workflow efficiency and maximize power of team-based care.
8. Reduce clerical burden and tame the EHR [EMR].
9. Support the physical and psychological health of the workforce.

Increasing evidence suggests that if an organization can improve its alignment with its key clinicians, then levels of burnout in the staff can be reduced by at least 10%–15%, because systems-level changes are enhanced. There are unfortunately few organizations like the Mayo Clinic that have made this a major driving factor for the leadership and that have achieved such success, and most health systems still tend to put most of the focus for change back on individual staff and clinical units.

Maslach (2017), the originator of much of the burnout research, now takes the view that burnout is more of a chronic situational process than an individual problem. She believes that social improvements in work environments can help prevent burnout and build engagement, noting that social improvements rely on the reciprocal relationships between colleagues. She has in recent years focused increasingly on developing a new model for a healthy workplace, much as is promoted at the Mayo Clinic. She has defined six factors of importance in this new model, which has a strong focus on increasing workers' engagement and the early detection and prevention of burnout. She believes that workers need to have the following:

1. A sustainable workload, which may include work-process redesign and increased resourcing
2. Individual choice and control, over decisions and workplace policies
3. Recognition and reward, for achievements and success
4. A supportive work community, with time to network and develop supportive work relationships
5. Fairness, respect, and social justice, throughout the workplace environment
6. Clear values and meaningful work, with the opportunity to see and share mutually important results and outcomes

Maslach has noted downsides to implementing person-only or individually focused interventions within workplaces. These include a tendency to "blame the victim" by concluding that burnout is caused by individual weakness, lack of resilience, or a clinical deficit, and burnout then tends to be viewed within a disability framework. Although this approach may make it possible to help the person cope better with situational stressors, the stressors themselves are not changed and may be ignored or seen as having less significance.

At a national level a potentially influential group has been formed by the National Academy of Medicine (2017a, 2017b) that aims to undertake a national collaborative effort to address aspects of the burnout problem. In particular, the group documented a series of well-defined research needs at both the organizational and the individual levels, but with a particular focus on the impact on patient outcomes. This works connects well with the recent publication by Shanafelt et al. (2017) describing the business case for investing in physician well-being. The authors concluded that improvement in physician well-being is possible and that investment is justified and return on investment is measurable, noting that addressing this issue is not just an ethical responsibility of organizations but fiscally responsible.

One approach that a number of organizations have taken in response to the burnout level findings is to give their physicians access to the Well-Being Index, a tool developed by the Mayo group (Shanafelt et al. 2014). The index is a nine-item validated questionnaire that anyone can take once for free on the commercial website at https://www.mededwebs.com/well-being-index. This interesting tool is not a measure of burnout, but it gives scores for physicians on several dimensions of distress, such as "meaning in work," "likelihood of burnout," "severe fatigue," "work-life integration, "risk for medical error," and "suicidal ideation." Scores are shown on a single dashboard and allow a single user to compare his or her scores against scores of all U.S. physicians who have filled out the questionnaire. As such, the Well-Being Index enables physicians to assess themselves, compared against colleagues, and then to focus on the problematic scoring areas, and, if they are using a licensed copy, to remeasure themselves and track their index score over time. The Well-Being Index comes with a series of good educational resources and relevant publications not just in the six dimensions of distress but in areas like health behavior, financial management, career and professional development, relationship and work-life balance, and malpractice and organizational and leadership issues. This sort of approach, where organizations give their physicians the power to self-assess, is likely to become common in future and is one of a number of creative interventions for which trials are being carried out to attempt to improve physician health and well-being, as discussed in Chapters 9 and 10 of this book.

So given that we know from the literature that burnout is usually organizationally driven, individuals can even so reduce their personal level of burnout by about the same amount as seen in the organizational change studies, in which burnout levels typically can be reduced by about 10% or more. What, then, can an individual physician do to improve his or her own situation?

There are many strategies, some of which Tina tried and others of which are discussed in Chapter 10, but they all have the same end point—to put balance and meaning back in the life of the individual physician. This is something that younger generations of physicians are likely better at than those in the baby-boomer generation. Millennials, currently ages 18–36, consisting of more than 60 million Americans and almost 20% of the medical workforce, are typically described as high maintenance with lots of expectations, but they are also high performing, especially if given the right environment with a combination of support and autonomy. They are notable for their commitment to, and interest in, friends, family, and hobbies, often ahead of work, and will hopefully drive changes in health systems and cultures that will, in the long run, reduce the amount of burnout. Recent research looking at highly successful commercial companies that attract a lot of younger workers shows that these companies frequently offer flexible scheduling, telecommuting options, paid sabbaticals, and paid volunteer days, as well as perks like massages and yoga, mindfulness, and fitness classes. All of these perks are, of course, excellent at reducing the likelihood of burnout and supporting life balance at an individual level and organizationally most certainly support the new model of work proposed by Maslach.

This younger generation is less affected by the single greatest current cause of burnout in most physicians—the EMR. As "digital natives," who have grown up in the age of the Internet and have never known what life is like without email, sophisticated search engines, and social media, they find the EMR and other health technologies and devices that are now rapidly infiltrating healthcare natural and easy to use. This is in contrast to many physicians, perhaps better thought of as "digital immigrants," who can well remember writing letters to friends and lovers, and who would still, secretly or otherwise, really prefer the old paper medical records, with their weighty tattered edges. Those days are gone, and although most health systems in the United States have switched over to EMRs in the past decade, an unexpected consequence, at least partially attributable to EMRs, has been the significant increase in burnout among physicians and other health professionals. Most health systems have taken the view that they just have to get the EMR implemented and that the users will somehow cope with it and learn as they go. Well physicians as a group are actually very good at adapting. They are intelligent, thoughtful, and flexible. Overall, they have adapted extremely well to some pretty dreadful EMRs that were primarily designed by engineers, many of which lack interfaces that integrate well into normal medical workflows and practices. As a consequence, the EMR for many physicians is a massive cause of stress. A recent time-and-motion study (Sinsky et al. 2016) of 57 physicians who were observed at their work for a total of 430 hours and who completed after-hours diaries showed that they only spent 27% of their total time on direct face time with patients. In contrast, 37% of their daily work time, not including 1–2 hours each evening, was spent on EMRs. This dramatic reduction in direct time to spend with patients, in the setting of increased work hours catching up with EMR activities, has in many cases led directly to the disillusionment and exhaustion that are key symptoms of burnout.

It is only in the past few years that the importance of this unexpected consequence has been recognized. We now know, as happened with Tina, that physicians have to be helped, with extra training and better documentation support, to be able to use the EMR without needing to either reduce their time with patients or exhaust themselves. Just as Tina suggested, efforts need to be made to take away from physicians the new and extra time-consuming busywork involved in maintaining an EMR, often related to administrative or financial functions. This may involve redesigning clinic workflows and increasing the amount of data input done by patients and during the rooming process undertaken by support staff. It is sad that it has taken such a long time for this realization to sink in across the health care environment, and sadder still that this need is not yet widely understood. There is now at last in many hospitals and clinics more attention being paid to the need for continuous training and updates on how to use these remarkably sophisticated software EMR packages, with their extraordinarily complicated and diverse functions.

The final issue of importance in Tina's case is her strength and resilience, a topic that will be discussed in more detail in Chapter 10. *Resilience* has been defined by Luthar et al. (2000) as the ability of an individual to maintain personal and social stability despite adversity. Beresin et al. (2016) have described how over time this conceptualization of resilience has moved away from considering it as a personality trait to thinking of it as a process that can be linked to a skill set that can be learned. They noted that resilience comprises two complementary activities, both preventive and corrective, by which individuals both actively resist adversity and cope effectively in traumatic situations. Tina showed a great deal of resilience in both these areas, with her capacity to make changes and to grow stronger within her workplace environment, and secondarily to respond to stress and bounce back in response to added challenges in her workplace. A number of studies have examined the factors that underpin this broader concept of resilience and the reasons some individuals are resilient, yet others are not. Epstein and Krasner (2013) noted that key issues are the capacity for mindfulness, limit setting, self-monitoring, and attitudes that promote healthy engagement with (instead of withdrawal from) work challenges:

> Cultivating the specific skills, habits, and attitudes that promote resilience is possible for medical students and practicing clinicians alike. Resilience-promoting programs should also strive to build community among clinicians and other members of the health care workforce. Just as patient safety is the responsibility of communities of practice, so is clinician well-being and support. Finally, it is in the self-interest of health care institutions to support the efforts of all members of the health care workforce to enhance their capacity for resilience; it will increase quality of care while reducing errors, burnout, and attrition. (p. 301)

When we look back at Tina's experience, it's evident that there were a number of organizational changes being implemented in her clinic that gave her and her colleagues more help and improved feelings of control and alignment with the clinic goals. She became involved in these changes and, in a healthy way, did exactly what Epstein and Krasner suggested by becoming engaged with her work challenges, rather than withdrawing from them as she had done initially. As a resilient individual she also made numerous individual changes in her personal life, achieving more balance and devoting more time for her family as well as focusing on her physical fitness. She improved her marriage and worked with her husband on resolving his fears about her physical health and her recovery from breast cancer. In her work life she specifically spent time training herself to use the clinic EMR better and enlisted others to help her with some of her data input, so that she could both keep better notes and keep the notes current without needing to write them on nights and weekends, when she deserved to have free time with her husband and family.

References

American Medical Association: STEPS Forward. Creating the organizational foundation for joy in medicine. 2018a. Available at: https://www.stepsforward.org/modules/joy-in-medicine. Accessed April 10, 2018.

American Medical Association: STEPS Forward. Physician wellness: preventing resident and fellow burnout. 2018b. Available at: https://www.stepsforward.org/modules/physician-wellness. Accessed April 10, 2018.

American Medical Association: STEPS Forward. Preventing physician burnout. 2018c. Available at: https://www.stepsforward.org/modules/physician-burnout. Accessed April 10, 2018.

Beresin EV, Milligan TA, Balon R, et al: Physician wellbeing: a critical deficiency in resilience education and training. Acad Psychiatry 40(1):9–12, 2016 26691141

Blue Ridge Academic Health Group: The hidden epidemic: the moral imperative for academic health centers to address health professionals' well-being. Report 22, Winter 2017–18. Available at: http://whsc.emory.edu/blueridge/publications/archive/blue-ridge-winter2017-2018.pdf. Accessed March 7, 2018.

Bohman B, Dyrbye L, Sinsky CA, et al: Physician well-being: the reciprocity of practice efficiency, culture of wellness, and personal resilience. NEJM Catalyst, August 7, 2017. Available at: https://catalyst.nejm.org/physician-well-being-efficiency-wellness-resilience. Accessed March 7, 2018.

Dyrbye LN, West CP, Satele D, et al: Burnout among U.S. medical students, residents, and early career physicians relative to the general U.S. population. Acad Med 89(3):443–451, 2014 24448053

Epstein RM, Krasner MS: Physician resilience: what it means, why it matters, and how to promote it. Acad Med 88(3):301–303, 2013 23442430

Luthar SS, Cicchetti D, Becker B: The construct of resilience: a critical evaluation and guidelines for future work. Child Dev 71(3):543–562, 2000 10953923

Maslach C: Burnout: what it is, how to address it. Keynote presentation presented at the Keys to Physician Wellness Conference. San Francisco, CA, August 24, 2017

Maslach C, Jackson S: The measurement of experienced burnout. Journal of Organizational Behavior 2:99–113, 1981

Medscape: Lifestyle report 2017. 2017. Available at: https://www.medscape.com/sites/public/lifestyle/2017. Accessed January 19, 2018.

National Academy of Medicine: Action Collaborative on Clinician Well-Being and Resilience, 2017a. Available at: https://nam.edu/initiatives/clinician-resilience-and-well-being. Accessed March 7, 2018.

National Academy of Medicine: Burnout among health care professionals: a call to explore and address this underrecognized threat to safe, high quality care. Discussion paper, 2017b. Available at: https://nam.edu/burnout-among-health-care-professionals-a-call-to-explore-and-address-this-underrecognized-threat-to-safe-high-quality-care. Accessed January 19, 2018.

Rothenberger DA: Physician burnout and well-being: a systematic review and framework for action. Dis Colon Rectum 60(6):567–576, 2017 28481850

Shanafelt TD, Noseworthy JH: Executive leadership and physician well-being: nine organizational strategies to promote engagement and reduce burnout. Mayo Clin Proc 92(1):129–146, 2017 27871627

Shanafelt TD, Kaups KL, Nelson H, et al: An interactive individualized intervention to promote behavioral change to increase personal well-being in US surgeons. Ann Surg 259(1):82–88, 2014

Shanafelt TD, Hasan O, Dyrbye LN, et al: Changes in burnout and satisfaction with work-life balance in physicians and the general US working population between 2011 and 2014. Mayo Clin Proc 90(12):1600–1613, 2015 26653297

Shanafelt T, Goh J, Sinsky C: The business case for investing in physician well-being. JAMA Intern Med 177(12):1826–1832, 2017 28973070

Sinsky C, Colligan L, Li L, et al: Allocation of physician time in ambulatory practice: a time and motion study in 4 specialties. Ann Intern Med 165(11):753–760, 2016 27595430

Stanford Medicine: WellMD: Stanford Wellness Framework. 2017. Available at: https://wellmd.stanford.edu. Accessed January 20, 2018.

The Second Victim

"**I CAN'T BELIEVE IT.** How did he die? What did he do?"

Dr. Julia Stuart sat down and took a deep breath to calm herself before continuing the phone conversation. She twisted the phone cord around her perfectly manicured fingers, playing with it constantly as if it were a set of rosary beads that somehow gave her the confidence to continue. She looked out of the window of her office, blankly, not focusing on anything, and thought about Tom, her friend and medical colleague, whom she had been planning on seeing later on that Friday evening for a social drink with a group of mutual friends. But Tom would not be there this Friday or any other evening ever again.

The phone conversation with the police officer continued, and Dr. Stuart rapidly agreed to meet with him in person to be interviewed about her friend and roommate's apparent suicide, if only to get him off the line and to give herself a moment to think by herself. She buzzed the front desk of her office and asked her receptionist to cancel all her other patients for the day. She was in no state to help others and needed some time for herself to think.

She looked around her office. Everything seemed so normal. A conventional geneticist's room with a loaded bookcase, pictures, and framed professional certificates on the walls; her neatly organized desk and computer; and of course the comfortable grouping of leather armchairs that she used to see her patients, explore their backgrounds, and counsel them about the many genetic disorders that afflicted them. All very normal, but somehow different and changed through the shock of Tom's death, and the loss of her closest friend. Absentmindedly she opened her bag and took out her makeup case so that she could start repairing her eyes, ruined by the recent copious tears. Why on earth had he killed himself? Should she, as a physician and friend, have been able to pick up how he felt and prevented this tragedy? What had led this brilliant young anesthesiologist to inject himself with the anesthetic propofol? Had he really been trying to kill himself, or was his an accidental overdose? If so, how had she missed seeing that he was presumably an addict, when she thought she knew him so well? Was she herself guilty of missing some signs from him? Could she have somehow helped prevent this? The feelings of confusion, shock, and even guilt distressed her massively.

As Julia gradually calmed down from the initial shock of hearing about Tom's death, she started thinking about him and the friendship she had had with him. They had both joined the faculty at the university at the same time, a year previously, and met at the orientation sessions. She was a new assistant professor of pediatric genetics, and he was in the same role in anesthesiology. They communicated well and shared a mutual interest in trying to learn the archaic rules and requirements for academic merit and promotion that seemed to be essential components of their new positions as clinical educators at the top-notch university. As they were both new to the city, it was not surprising that they soon became friends, with similar outside interests and over time an increasingly wide social network of young single professionals. They decided to rent a house with one other medical colleague and soon settled into a comfortable lifestyle as colleagues and, she had thought, increasingly close friends.

Tom was slim, casual, and usually neatly dressed when not in his scrubs or gym gear. He had blond, slightly too long hair and a boyish look that she had always found attractive. He was at times stressful to be with. She reflected about how Tom could be the life and soul of a party but at other times unaccountably absent or missing, much of which she attributed to his long work hours. Julia sometimes wondered about whether he had relationships he just preferred to keep private to himself. She had heard rumors that he might be gay but had always ignored these stories. He had had several short relationships that never seemed to go anywhere, and one evening he told her about a long-term girlfriend who he said lived several states away, but then he never mentioned her again. He never showed any romantic interest in her, treating her almost like a sister, which was diffi-cult as she secretly wished he would make a pass at her so that their friend-ship might become more than that.

Her receptionist let her know the police had arrived at her office. Her heart was racing as she let the officers enter her room. She was trying to maintain her composure despite feeling anxious about what they were about to tell her. Julia usually had an air of confidence with her tall and fit figure and long blond hair lying loose across her shoulders. She looked the part of a true professional with her navy pencil-style skirt and taupe silk blouse all coordinated with her silk scarf. Her white lab coat with her name proudly stitched on the left pocket hung on a hook by the door. She was somewhat relieved that the police had advised her to stay at work, rather than go back to her home, where the coroner and his team were busy collecting evidence. The thought of what Tom must have looked like when he was found sent shivers down her body. Tom being put into a white zippered body bag to be taken to the morgue was such a gruesome thought. She was glad she had avoided that scene.

"What happened?" Julia asked the officers. "What did he do?"

"It looks like suicide but we can't be certain of course until the coroner has done his investigation. He was in the bathroom with a propofol IV in his arm. It looks like he put it in himself, and from the look of his arms, he had been using needles for a long time. We don't know the exact time of death, but he was probably gone several hours when we got to him. Can we ask you some questions about Tom?"

Julia was shocked and confused at the comment about needle marks. She felt nauseated. How could he have hidden this from her?

"We looked around his room," the police officers continued. "We found a locked suitcase under his bed full of propofol vials, needles, and IV setups. It looks to us like he was using drugs for a long time. It seems he was likely an addict. Were you aware of this?"

Julia gasped and couldn't stop herself from bursting into tears. "No, that can't be possible. Not Tom. I can't believe it. We were close friends. We saw each other every day. He had ups and downs, but I don't understand. And he was doing really well at work. I presume you know he is—he was—an anesthesiologist here at the med center."

The female police officer continued gently. "We realize that. We're looking for some more background information before we inform his family. Did you know about his large supply of vials of drugs, needles, and syringes as well as drip equipment in his room? We had a quick look in his car and found more IV equipment in the trunk, complete with labels from the hospital here. It looks like he was regularly taking home supplies."

By now Julia was completely shocked and taken aback. She sat rigidly in one of her armchairs, just like her most traumatized patients during counseling sessions, almost at a complete loss for words, having to absorb a dreadful new truth. Denial about what was happening was screaming in her brain. How could she have missed all this? How had she not noticed something? What had been going on? What sort of a physician was she that she had been unable to recognize Tom as being at risk?

Over the next few days and weeks, Julia kept asking herself these same questions. She found herself more frequently double-checking medication dosages and clinical information that she knew well. She became more uncertain about her whole knowledge base and less confident in her interactions with her patients. She wanted to talk to her colleagues about this but felt unable to do so. She feared they would see her as weak. Oddly there seemed to be a cone of silence where Tom was concerned. She knew other colleagues and friends were upset, but there seemed to be a determined push by almost everyone to just keep on with their normal lives, at work and at home, and not to talk about how they all felt.

Six months later Julia was sitting in the break room at her clinic midmorning drinking what she thought must be about her fourth cup of coffee of the day. She adjusted her sweater, which she absently noticed was too big for her. She had little interest in food and had lost 20 pounds. She knew she should get back to the gym, but she couldn't stir up the energy or the motivation. She was beginning to hope her patients would not show up at times. She was tired of seeing patients and knew she no longer was empathizing with them as she used to. Several of her patients had recently commented on the recent changes in her and how she seemed to be distant and on edge. One of them had managed to upset her quite seriously by saying she thought that Julia, the doctor, looked worse than the patient herself, and Julia had ended up in tears after the session and left the clinic early in distress, causing problems by her sudden absence and abandoning a full schedule of patients.

Still, she reflected that this event a week ago seemed to be forgotten, and she had returned the following day with nothing being said to her. She knew that as long as her patient load remained reasonably light she could cope a little longer. She knew her colleagues were worried about her because most of them had been avoiding her—not surprising, really, given how much she had been exploding in their direction when they annoyed her. They now almost seemed embarrassed to meet up with her. She noticed that if she kept to her room as much as possible and avoided the public areas of the clinic, she could keep out of their way and avoid any confrontations.

She found she was obsessing about Tom and the awful aftermath of his death. She just couldn't stop these thoughts and was constantly preoccupied with all that had happened. It seemed impossible to clear the memories from her mind and focus on anything else.

She thought about all her feelings at the time: pain, sadness, guilt, regret; frustration at unknowns; fear as she carried on working and living almost like a zombie in the weeks following his suicide. She remembered the many meetings—small and large—and the memorials and the funeral—most of which she found unhelpful personally because she was enveloped in her own silent and secret guilt and grief. The official communications, which she knew had to be disseminated, sometimes acted like an extra knife twisting, making her guilt and sadness worse. There was all the discussion about Tom's death—was it deliberate suicide, or was he just taking a large amount of propofol, an anesthetic, to try to sleep and get some peace with himself? Could this have been a mistake and just one bad decision and miscalculation of the propofol dosage? Many of his colleagues and friends were still trying to argue it was all a mistake, but the note that was beside his body, saying good-bye to her as one of several named friends, argued against this. Julia knew that this was no accidental overdose and that Tom had killed himself deliberately.

She thought about the weeks following his death. Of the frustration and hidden anger in his department and among his colleagues and friends. Of the stigma attached to his suicide, which was connected by some to vague hints about his supposedly gay lifestyle. Of the need to cover his workload. Of, in particular, all the night call that he had volunteered for that others now had to do at short notice. Of the lack of acknowledgment of his loss. She felt frustrated with the health system itself for its poor official communications about Tom's death. It was always easy to make the institution a target, and she could see how that had happened when the CEO tried to downplay Tom's death in public. It had been explained to her by the public relations people that it was "in everyone's best interest to downplay" suicides. The health system had policies in place to minimize the possibility of what she now knew was called "suicide contagion," or what she had always thought of as copycat suicides or suicide attempts, which she had seen a few times in her career. Unfortunately, from Julia's perspective, this made it even more difficult to talk about how she felt, because there seemed to be a big silent cloak that had been thrown over the institution that prevented such discussion. At times it was as if Tom had never existed.

Of course, she realized that it wasn't true that the health system didn't make efforts to help its staff recognize the signs of burnout and suicide risk factors. She knew that the sudden interest that the health system leaders were showing in physician wellness was no coincidence. She had gone to one of the workshops on burnout but had found it unhelpful—what good was learning about yoga and time management going to be to her? She had even been asked to join a committee to examine the professional climate of the institution, which she realized was an attempt to prevent any more suicides. She declined because she didn't feel up to participating since she was focused only on keeping herself going, keeping up with her patient load, and moving to a new home. She could recall being involved in discussions about suicide prevention, and although she knew this was important and she wanted the topic to be raised, she found herself getting angry and took the discussion very personally, as if she had failed. She knew in her head that not all suicides are preventable and that each person sees differing aspects of an individual at risk, and not the whole picture, but the logic of these thoughts somehow didn't stop her angry and frustrated feelings. She couldn't stay in the house where Tom had died and felt anxious and upset anytime she had to go there. Luckily she had friends who had offered her a short-term room so she had never had to sleep in the house again after his death, but it had been painful going back there to move her belongings in the subsequent weeks.

So why was Dr. French, her rather formal but kindly mentor and senior pediatric colleague, suddenly appearing in the break room and making himself some coffee? He didn't usually do that, and they hadn't met for what should have been regular monthly mentoring sessions for at least 3 months as she had made excuses to miss them.

"Julia, I'm worried about you and want to have a private discussion with you if you don't mind. Would it be OK if we went to your office since we both seem to have some free time right now?"

Julia instantly bristled and responded angrily. "What do you mean by that? I'm fine. There is nothing wrong with me. I can't believe you said that. Are you trying to harass me or something? I have no intention of talking to you or anybody else about myself. I'm able to cope, and how I manage myself is up to me." At which stage she stalked out of the room and went to seclude herself in her office. Dr. French sighed but, with persistence, followed her down the corridor and into her room.

"Look, Julia. You must know something is wrong with you and that you've not been performing well here in the clinic in recent months. There have been several patient complaints about your attitude, and the staff all feel like they have to walk on eggshells whenever you're around because you get upset and angry at minor problems. This just cannot go on. It's something we have to discuss."

Julia slumped in a chair and turned away, looking into the corner of the room as if she might find an escape hatch there. Dr. French continued in a caring tone.

"Julia, you haven't been the same since the tragedy of your friend killing himself. Quite frankly none of us have been the same, such has been the impact of his suicide on all the faculty and students here. But I understand you were a close friend of his, as well as a roommate, and it must have been dreadfully difficult for you."

Julia turned to look at Dr. French as her tears fell gently down her face. Dr. French gave her some time to recover and dry her eyes with some strategically placed tissues that were usually meant for her patients. Then he continued: "I don't want to be too intrusive, but you need to understand that I'm here at our departmental chairman's request to see if we can work something out and get you some help if you'll accept that. Our chair is really concerned about you, as am I, and is worried that if this goes on you will start making mistakes and be unfit to practice. In fact, he's so concerned about you that he has already consulted with the chair of the hospital faculty well-being committee, a psychiatrist who has been treating faculty and staff from all over our region for years. The psychiatrist's advice was for us to talk to you informally and try and persuade you to see a colleague of his who works outside of our hospital system. He said, from our chair's description, that it sounded like you were anxious and depressed and may have what is now being called second victim syndrome. He said that a number of other faculty have ended up having counseling following your friend's suicide and that the impact has been really widespread. Much more so than you or I would ever suspect."

Julia listened intently, starting to feel somewhat reassured. It seemed to her that she was not alone. That others had also been affected. But they couldn't have felt as guilty as she felt. They couldn't have been responsible for missing the signs of Tom's addiction, and his eventual suicide, like she felt she was.

Dr. French continued: "I think you really should talk about it with someone. I know we can't insist on this, but I think it would be helpful. Would you like to tell me what has been happening? I promise you the details will all be confidential. We're all really worried about you and want to see you back to how you used to be."

Julia burst into tears and responded angrily. "I can't believe it's come to this. None of this is my fault. If Tom hadn't killed himself, all would be fine and I wouldn't feel so guilty. And now it sounds like you think I'm not coping. I know you're trying to be kind, but I feel like such a failure. I keep feeling that I'm guilty for what happened with Tom. I know that I should have been able to stop what happened. I can see that I missed a whole series of hints that he gave to me. I was his best friend here in town, and I don't think he had many other friends elsewhere, what with his family abandoning him years ago. I just feel so guilty, so guilty. I am constantly thinking of him. Look here, on my phone, here are some photos we took at a departmental dinner just a week before he died. Look how sad he looks compared with everyone else. I just can't stop looking at the photos. See, there he is in another one—sad again. Why didn't I see this before he killed himself? Why didn't I do something?"

Julia got up from her chair and walked around the room, agitated and distressed, wringing her hands, absently picking up a picture of her family from a sideboard. "Look. I have a family who loves me. Tom had no one except me and some other colleagues here. And I didn't pay enough attention to him. Obviously it now seems that he was an addict for several years—that came out clearly enough in the coroner's investigation—and that he had managed to hide his addiction and his distress from everyone, even me, his roommate, the person who felt closest to him. I just know that if I were able to go back to before he died, I could have prevented it, and prevented all the distress and awful goings-on that have happened here as a result of his death. Why didn't I do that? I can't believe how I missed everything, and yet I know I didn't. I know now, when I'm really honest with myself, that I did see that something was wrong but that I didn't want to admit it, and didn't want to ask him about it. And even if I had consciously thought about confronting him about it, how would I have done that? He was a friend and a colleague. They don't tell you how to have those sorts of discussions in medical school."

She sat down again and cried some more, but more gently this time. "I should have confronted him about it. I'm the guilty one. I did see that he had all those odd mood swings—sometimes happy and the absolute life of the party, but more often anxious and on edge, usually before he went to work. I can see now how he was getting hold of his drugs at work, and why he loved working long hours, weekends and nights, because it was at work that he could find the narcotic tablets and vials he took himself. He loved being at work because he could get high there, and that's why he always used to like doing the shifts other doctors wouldn't do. He was relatively unsupervised then and could get hold of the drugs he needed with relatively few nurses or doctors around to check on him. That was one of the reasons we never started having a relationship, although I was certainly keen enough—he just never seemed to be that interested in me. Now I know, not only was he hiding his sexual preference, but that he had another mistress – his drugs. And I couldn't see it at the time."

Julia looked up at Dr. French, who was listening intently, and continued. "You know, I think I really did know what was happening. I've just been afraid to admit it to myself until now. He was always very secretive about what was in his room, and would sometimes go into the bathroom for hours at a time, with no good excuse. I think he must have been putting himself on an IV at those times. And now that I'm being honest with myself, I did see him with some vials of drugs in his car on a couple of occasions, but he just laughed my query off, saying they were for his research project. I knew that wasn't true, but I was afraid to confront him. Living in the same house as him, even though we sometimes didn't see each other much for several days if we were on opposite shifts, I realized that there was a problem with him, but I just didn't want to admit it to myself or to think about asking him about it. After all, I think I was a little bit in love with him, and I just didn't want to rock the boat and potentially damage any relationship I might eventually have with him. What a fool. Look what I've done."

Julia looked like she had almost completely run out of steam, so intense was her guilt and her preoccupation with Tom's suicide. She stopped talking and looked down at her shoes, exhausted, sad, and guilt-ridden.

"Julia—I don't think you need to feel as guilty as you do. After all, it was ultimately Tom's illness and his way of coping that led to his death."

This seemingly gentle response seemed to startle Julia, and she sat up suddenly, upset and distressed. "No. I should have prevented it. I just didn't know how to approach him and talk to him about what was going on with him. I knew deep down that there was something bad going on with him; it just didn't click that he could be an addict. He was such a warm charismatic man much of the time that I refused to contemplate that he had a problem. You know, I've never told anyone this, but I did think of talking to him about how he was, about 2 weeks before he died. I found him in the kitchen of our home one morning early, and he was really quite confused and seemed to be intoxicated, yet I knew he didn't drink and he had on several occasions expressed intense anger towards addicts who took illegal drugs. I took his arm and went to try and take his pulse and see how he was, and he suddenly became furious with me. Very angry and defensive. Way out of line. It was really awkward and embarrassing, and it was clear he wanted to make sure I couldn't see his arms to take his pulse. I thought it was very odd, and he just ran out of the room and went to his bedroom, and never mentioned the incident again, except to go out of his way to tell me the following day that he felt fine. He always used to wear long-sleeve shirts, even in surgery under his scrubs, because he said he had dermatitis and was very sensitive about the look it gave his arms, but his reaction was way more than any local embarrassment. I know now that he wore the long-sleeve shirts to cover up needle marks on his arms, and if only I had tried to check him out properly when he was obviously intoxicated, I would have discovered his needle track marks and would have been able to try and help him. If only I had not let my suspicions go after that incident, he might be alive today. If only I had just used the most basic clinical reasoning that all physicians are trained to use, I would have realized what was going on and could have talked to him about it. But I was afraid to admit I had seen the signs—his mood changes, the drugs in his car, the intoxication, his odd hours at work. And anyway how could I have approached him about something like this? I have no idea how to approach friends or colleagues who may be unwell in this way. That would be so hard. It's just not something I've ever thought I would need to think about."

By now Julia was slowing down. Less angry. Less reactive. No longer crying but really wrung out emotionally. Dr. French tried to persuade her to see a counselor, but she refused outright, saying that she knew how to handle herself and would be fine. Finally, as a compromise, she agreed to go online and do the anonymous depression self-assessment that the hospital well-being committee had developed. And she agreed to meet up with Dr. French again as a check-in in a couple of weeks.

The following day she had two patients who canceled, so she suddenly had a free hour. She had thought a lot about the discussion with Dr. French and was intrigued by his idea that she should take the hospital online depression self-assessment. She knew about the questionnaire because once a year all physicians received a reminder about it from the chair of the well-being committee, suggesting that they take it and emphasizing that it was completely anonymous. She ran through her old email to find it and reread the invitation to take the "confidential stress and depression questionnaire."

> Dear Colleague,
>
> Today I write to you not only as the chair of the Hospital Medical Staff Well-Being Committee, but as a colleague who cares deeply about the health and well-being of everyone associated with Health System. I am pleased to remind you about an important service offered to the medical students, residents, and faculty, developed and managed by the Medical Staff Well-Being Committee: a program to confidentially screen, identify and offer treatment to those among us suffering from depression and other problems that may interfere with social, academic, and personal functioning.
>
> Using the link here, you will be taken to a secure, confidential website to complete a simple, brief questionnaire instrument called the Stress and Depression Questionnaire. This will take about 10 minutes to complete. You

will be asked to choose a User ID and a password to log in. Please follow the instructions provided on the website. The User ID and password will be the only two pieces of information required in returning your completed questionnaire. Please be assured that since your responses and all other information you communicate through the website will be identified only with the User ID you assign to yourself, **your identity will be fully protected**. You can also access the survey and view further information about the questionnaire through the Medical Staff Well-Being website.

Within 24–48 hours of submission, a trained mental health counselor will review each questionnaire submitted. This counselor will then send you a personal response **although the counselor will have no idea who they are replying to**. The response will include an assessment and, when appropriate, recommendations for further evaluation or follow-up. You will then have the opportunity to communicate online with the mental health counselor if you wish, at which stage you can continue to communicate anonymously, or you can choose to tell them who you are. Alternatively, you may meet with the counselor who works at the hospital in the employee assistance program face-to-face, if that is your preference. The goal will be to help those with stress, depression, or other mental health issues affecting functioning to get help. There is no reason to break your anonymity with this program if you do not want to.

While completing the online questionnaire and participating in this program is completely voluntary and confidential, I *strongly urge everyone to complete the questionnaire*. I believe we have an obligation not only to help those individuals who suffer from depression and related problems, but also to understand the scope and nature of these problems throughout our community and we are interested to know what is the size of this particular problem within our community. This problem will be best addressed through a public health approach, and that will require the cooperation of **everyone**.

In the same spirit of professionalism that characterizes our dedication to the sick and the prevention of illness in our patients, I ask you for the sake of your health and well-being, and that of your friends, coworkers, and colleagues, to take a few minutes of your time to complete and submit this questionnaire.

Warmest personal regards,

Jeremy Store, M.D.
Chair, Hospital Medical Staff, Health System Well-Being Committee

Julia decided that she had nothing to lose by at least completing this anonymous self-assessment and that it would be interesting to see how she scored, and what the response from the counselor was like. So she made up an ID and password and started to complete the questionnaire. She was pleased to see that it really did seem completely confidential. She was asked to put in her gender, her age to the nearest decade, and whether she was a medical student, resident, or attending physician, but no other information about herself. She felt confident that she would not be able to be identified from the hundred or more female physicians in her age range who worked in the hospital.

She started reading and responding to the questions and was surprised at how specific they were. She answered "never" to items that asked if she had thoughts about taking her own life, had planned ways of taking her life, or had done things to hurt herself. In the next section, though, she found herself answering either "often" or "sometimes" to a series of questions about depression that she recognized from one of the questionnaires she sometimes used with patients who she thought might be depressed. In the next section she pondered for some time on how to respond to a question that asked if she was "feeling intensely anxious, feeling intensely angry, feeling hopeless, feeling desperate or feeling out of control." She decided she really should be as honest as possible, as this sentence described exactly how she felt, so she answered "most or all of the time." The final section of the questionnaire asked her a series of questions about her use of drugs and alcohol, and since she drank little and had never used any illegal or painkilling drugs, except for the occasional use of ibuprofen for headaches, she replied in the negative. The whole online questionnaire actually took her about 15 minutes to complete, longer than predicted, mainly because the section on depression had really made her think and had slowed her up. Here she recognized that she was completing a well-validated, scientifically researched set of questions on depression that she used with her patients, and she knew that she was answering in a way that would lead to her being concerned if one of her patients had answered like she had. Was it really possible that she had developed depression herself and just not recognized this consciously? Was this what Dr. French and her colleagues were seeing in her? She wondered how the psychologist who saw her results would respond to her.

Julia decided to wait 24 hours before logging back into the system using her anonymous user ID and password, and when she did so she found a note waiting for her:

Counselor Name: Amy Brown, Ph.D., Director of Counseling Services
Health System Employee Assistance Program
Counselor Address: Newport Building, First Floor
Tel: Counselor Direct Line (1-916-321-5656)

My name is Amy Brown and I'm a counselor at the Health System Employee Assistance Program. I have reviewed your responses to the Stress and Depression Questionnaire and am particularly concerned that you have recently been feeling intensely anxious, and angry, and feeling hopeless, and feeling desperate or out of control. You also say in the questionnaire that you often feel depressed and that these feelings are making your life very difficult. I am also concerned that you scored 15 on the Personal Health Questionnaire section of the screening, suggesting that you may well have clinically significant depression. It is good that you do not report overuse of drugs or alcohol.

I believe I can help you find relief, and I hope that you will contact me to set up a time we can get together within the next day or two.

If you would rather talk to me without coming in or identifying yourself, we can continue to exchange messages on this website. You can respond to me by clicking on the "Dialogue" button below, and I promise I will respond to your message over the website as quickly as I can. You can generally expect to hear back from me within 24 hours, although over the weekend or during holiday periods, it may take me a little longer to get back to you. If you provided an email address in the questionnaire you submitted, you will receive an email message when I have responded to your Dialogue note. If you contact me through this website, please make sure you keep a record of your User ID and password so you can log back on to get my response.

If you prefer, we can also talk by phone; just give me a call at the number listed above. You will not need to identify yourself by name unless you want to.

If you are in crisis, please call me. If you are unable to reach me, please refer to the Welcome page of this website for other numbers to call.

Please do let me hear from you. I think I can be of help and would like to see you as soon as possible.

Julia sat back and looked out of her window, thinking deeply. Nothing in the note surprised her, except possibly the obvious level of concern that the counselor was showing. She had done a lot of thinking in the past 24 hours. The meeting with Dr. French, and then the experience of completing the online wellness questionnaire, had had a real impact. She had started to realize that she had changed in the past 6 months, and she was thankful for her decision to answer the questionnaire honestly and not "fake good" as she knew many people did. But a score of 15 was significant, and above the cutoff score for depression, and she knew that really meant that she needed help. How should she respond to the counselor's email? How confidential was the whole process? She felt she needed some time to think, so she decided to take her time and try to find out more from the counselor.

Physician ID: "Female Professional"
To: Amy Brown, Ph.D., Director of Counseling Services
Health System Employee Assistance Program
Counselor Address: Newport Building, First Floor
Tel: Counselor Direct Line (1-916-321-5656)

Dear Amy: Thank you for your kind response, which I appreciate. I think you are right in what you say, and I understand the significance of my screening score of 15 on depression. I am very concerned about my confidentiality and whether seeking treatment may have any effect on my medical license and capacity to work here. Who might get to know about this? Will the Medical Board be notified?

"Female Professional"

Julia had a sleepless night. She just couldn't stop thinking about Amy's email and the obvious concern that Amy was showing. Was she really that unwell that a Ph.D. psychologist would be entreating her to connect with her—through the website, by phone, or in person? She finally gave up sleeping at 5 A.M. and got up. After making herself a steaming-hot cup of coffee, she decided she could wait no longer and logged in to the wellness website from her home laptop. There was a response from Dr. Brown already.

Counselor Name: Amy Brown, Ph.D., Director of Counseling Services
Health System Employee Assistance Program
Counselor Address: Newport Building, First Floor
Tel: Counselor Direct Line (1-916-321-5656)

Dear "Female Professional": Thank you for replying to me. It is good that you understand that you have a high depression score. I believe it would be helpful for you to either meet with me, or to allow me to help you arrange a referral to see a counselor or psychiatrist of your choice. I assure you that this process is entirely confidential and that even if you do decide to break your anonymity, that process will continue. I am unable to answer your question about your medical license because every situation is different, but my experience has been that our medical professionals who obtain treatment, and keep themselves well, are much less likely to be reported to the Medical Board because they have kept themselves well and any health problems they have do not ultimately affect their patient care, which is what the Medical Board is worried about.

As I said previously, I believe I can help you find relief, and I hope that you will contact me to set up a time we can get together within the next day or two. If you would rather talk to me without coming in or identifying yourself, we can continue to exchange messages on this website. If you prefer, we can also talk by phone; just give me a call at the number listed above. You will not need to identify yourself by name unless you want to.

If you are in crisis, please call me. If you are unable to reach me, please refer to the Welcome page of this website for other numbers to call.

Best wishes,
Amy Brown

Julia sat back and sipped her coffee. She knew she was going to have to make a decision sometime soon as to what she was going to do. After all, even if she did nothing, Dr. French was bound to follow up with her, and anyway she acknowledged now that she was feeling miserable, since she had started to think about herself honestly. If only Tom had not killed himself. If only she had picked up all the hints he had given before his suicide. If only she had approached him about his odd behaviors. If only she had not been so selfish and hoped that their relationship might go further than the friendship level. She knew that that was partly why she had been blinded to his behavior. So was it surprising that she felt so guilty? That it was at least partly her fault that he had died. She broke out of her guilty reverie and decided she had to make a decision. She couldn't stand the thought of many more sleepless nights.

Physician ID: "Female Professional"
To: Amy Brown, Ph.D., Director of Counseling Services
Health System Employee Assistance Program
Counselor Address: Newport Building, First Floor
Tel: Counselor Direct Line (1-916-321-5656)

Dear Amy: You have replied very quickly. Thank you. What you say makes sense and I know I need some help. I think I would like to see someone but I don't want this to be anyone who works for our Health System. I would like to see someone completely independent. Can you help with that?

"Female Professional"

At lunch the same day, Julia logged in again, to find a reply from Dr. Brown already posted.

Counselor Name: Amy Brown, Ph.D., Director of Counseling Services
Health System Employee Assistance Program
Counselor Address: Newport Building, First Floor
Tel: Counselor Direct Line (1-916-321-5656)

Dear "Female Professional": Thank you for following up. I am pleased that you want me to help you. The best option would be for us to meet in person. That will allow me to understand your situation better and work out with you what type of referral would be best for you. Regarding your question about the Medical Board, I phoned Dr. Store, who is a psychiatrist and chair of the Well-Being Committee, and he confirmed that there is no need for the Medical Board to know anything about you as long as there is no problem with the quality of your medical practice. He said that many physicians see psychiatrists for lots of different reasons, and noted that most of his outpatients are physicians, and that they work at other health systems as well as our own. So I hope that reassures you. Please do phone me or give me your contact information so we can set something up.

Best wishes, Amy Brown

Julia read the email with a feeling of relief. She still wasn't sure what would happen, but she knew she had to take some steps to help herself and to try to reduce her guilt feelings. She realized that the health system did have methods in place to help her, the healer, and not just the patients who attended for care. She liked Dr. French and was confident his motives for approaching her were good, and she felt she could trust Dr. Brown to arrange appropriate follow-up and treatment for her. She picked up the phone and dialed Dr. Brown's number.

Commentary

This case highlights several important issues: the impact of suicide on second victims, the internal and external responses of health systems to suicides of their physicians and potentially other staff, and the way these responses are oftentimes viewed by those close to the victims. It also demonstrates the difficulty that is sometimes seen in engaging physicians in psychiatric care and illustrates creative ways to do this.

Julia is a classic example of what is now being called a "second victim" of a major unexpected event, whether this be an unexpected death of a patient or colleague, a major clinical mistake or disaster, or, as an observer, a significant assault or traumatic event. In recent times in America the most obvious examples of such mass events are the 9/11 attack in New York and Washington, D.C., and the other terrorist- or gun-related mass disasters and attacks that have become all too common. These events all leave large numbers of second victims who are adversely affected, distressed, and traumatized. Such individuals often find it very hard to seek care, because it's easier to hide away and ignore personal hurt, often comparing themselves with others who were killed or maimed, and somehow not believing that their situation is serious enough to warrant attention.

In healthcare the importance of the second victim syndrome has only recently been recognized. Susan Scott, of the University of Missouri, has defined *second victims* as healthcare team members "involved in an unanticipated adverse patient event, in a medical error and/or a patient related injury and become victimized in the sense that the provider is traumatized by the event. Frequently, these individuals feel personally responsible for the patient outcome. Many feel as though they have failed the patient, second guessing their clinical skills and knowledge base" (Scott et al. 2009, p. 326).

In this case Julia was failed by her health system because she was left alone and not provided with extra emotional support after Tom's death to allow her, if she wished, to process her feelings. Her discussions with

Dr. French, some 6 months later, were helpful to her but would have been much more useful had they occurred months earlier. Second victim syndrome is a common disorder, most likely linked to burnout, and surveys have indicated that up to 40% of health staff at some time or other suffer from this. In most people the syndrome is self-limiting and the individuals affected recover as they gain support from colleagues and friends; however, a substantial minority, like Julia, have continuing symptoms and may progress to either burnout or depression. We know that second victim syndrome is important because it is associated with increased incidences of medical errors and absenteeism, worse clinical outcomes, and higher staff turnover. In Julia's case she noticed concerns about her knowledge base soon after Tom's death and then suffered increasing numbers of intrusive thoughts and regrets, before eventually developing full-blown depression after several months. At that stage, a few months after Tom's death, she had most of the biological symptoms of depression, including impaired attention, concentration, sleep, appetite, and mood, but even then did not recognize this illness in herself and had to be very slowly and gradually pulled into treatment. Some health systems, such as at the University of Missouri, now have detailed policies on how to care for the caregiver that include information on high-risk scenarios, common responses and symptoms, and the recovery stages. Recovery comprises six predictable stages, which are defined on the University of Missouri Health Care Web site as follows (University of Missouri Health Care 2018):

1. Chaos and accident response
2. Intrusive reflections
3. Restoring personal integrity
4. Enduring the inquisition
5. Obtaining emotional first aid
6. Moving on
   - Dropping out
   - Surviving
   - Thriving

The scenario shows how Julia felt about moving through all of these stages, but she only reached the substage of "surviving" in her attempt to move on, partly because she had not been able to reach out for support and partly because such support from her institution was lacking.

Some health systems are being very proactive in their response to second victims. The University of California, San Diego, is an example where a three-tier system has been developed to support staff. This model consists of, on the first level, local support on individual units, known as *code lavender*, from a caregiver support team, who constitute 10% of all staff, all of whom have received at least 8 hours of training from a psychologist, have a special marking on their badges, and attend monthly debriefing meetings. Second-level support makes available immediate debriefings for intense events. The third level of support consists of the employee assistance program and other more formal counseling and treatment interventions. Early results reported in 2017 by William Norcross, M.D., Director of the UC San Diego Physician Assessment and Clinical Education Program (http://www.paceprogram.ucsd.edu/), were very positive, with staff reporting a significant increase in their level of being "cared for" in the workplace and one staff suicide reportedly aborted. Dr. Norcross, in describing the code lavender intervention, called it a "culture shifting" intervention, and it has been very well received and is being disseminated throughout the institution with increased resourcing.

Julia also experienced a range of other symptoms and feelings that often affect survivors of tragedies. Clearly prevention messaging from a health system, while important, can be jarring for survivors of loss. Although such individuals want the topic to be raised, it has to be done well, and survivors who hear someone saying that an event was "preventable" tend to get angry and refer to themselves as having failed. In this instance, Tom's suicide may have been preventable, and it is evident that Julia tortured and blamed herself for not picking up on his symptoms and signs.

This is a normal reaction, although Julia most certainly was not seeing the whole picture as it related to Tom and was only able to pick up, consciously and unconsciously, a few components or hints of his drug abuse and potential dangerousness to himself. Survivors frequently suffer considerable frustration with their institutions and with the many unknowns. It is often unclear what has been said, if much, to the family of the victim, and there may initially be uncertainty about whether the death was an accident or suicide, which further complicates matters for everyone. In some respects the easiest target for any staff members in this situation is the institution itself, and so it is important for relevant leaders to be as open and up-front about institutional responses as possible. One way that individuals such as Julia do respond is to organize and advocate at their institution, in both the short and the long term, and supporting their efforts to do this is sensible and usually useful. It is possible to, for instance, form committees for well-being; present well-being materials in the orientations for new staff, medical students, and residents; develop and present workshops; and create other educational offerings on fatigue and burnout. These are all potentially positive responses to the suicide that suggest that second victims have moved to the thriving level.

The issue of institutional responses to suicide of an inpatient, which can be devastating, is important and has been studied. Indeed, such a suicide is defined in a formal way by the Joint Commission, which accredits hospitals and health systems, as a "reviewable sentinel event" that has to be examined by a "root cause analysis" within a 45-day period to identify possible causes or underlying factors that led to the event. Frameworks for immediate, short-term, and long-term responses to an inpatient suicide have been published (Ballard et al. 2008) and form a good guide for health systems to respond to the sort of tragedy described in this case. Such an institutional response in the short term, using Ballard et al.'s 2008 guideline, should ideally cover the following relevant key areas:

- Initial communication and administrative actions, with response teams and leaders designated and notifications made to families, staff, legal and regulatory bodies, and potentially the media
- Clinical assessment/management of other individuals at risk of suicide, as well as staff and patient responses and possible need for early debriefing
- Environment of care, including ensuring safety of locked areas and interactions with police and medical examiner officers, and the impact on staff and patients
- Policy and procedures, with the use of an emergency response checklist and possible implementation of short-term geographic or movement restrictions to ensure environmental safety

Another institutional response to the issue of physician suicide that is especially creative, and which was helpful for Julia, is the development and implementation of self-assessment tools. Why are these tools necessary, and why do physicians frequently not recognize that they need help for depression, anxiety, and substance disorders in particular? Julia is a good example of someone who has a fairly classical hand of symptoms of depression, yet she just tried to soldier on with her work and her life, and she didn't want to seek treatment. She was used to handling problems herself and not asking for help. There are many reasons for this, and they will be seen throughout the cases in this book, but this is a good time to look broadly at how many physicians develop and live throughout their life span, to try to understand them and, better, what drives them.

It is useful to think developmentally of five stages of a physician's life and look at the pressures and stresses that affect them:

- *Childhood/adolescence.* Frequently physicians come from high-performing families, often with physician parents, where work expectations and commitment are substantial, especially among Asian ethnic groups. Enjoyment of life and having fun are sublimated to work, which takes priority and for which rewards are gained. Success in academics and other competitive activities is often more important than success in friendships and relationships.

- *Young adulthood.* Here there are profound performance demands, intolerance of failure or even mediocrity, and delayed gratification for enjoyable pursuits. Career decisions to enter medical school are often made in high school, and potential medical students often start improving their résumé by increasing their community activities and volunteering, shadowing experts, and devoting more time toward their potential career. This all takes precedence over relationships, travel, and often fun, and the importance of delayed gratification, with less enjoyable activities and fewer financial rewards than they see their friends receiving, becomes entrenched early.

- *Medical school and residency.* These phases of education and training entail 8–12 years of hard labor and the worry for many of massively increasing personal debt. The high costs incurred (averaging $170,000 per qualifying medical student in 2017) put most medical students behind their non–medical student friends in the capacity to buy houses or cars, travel, or start families. More delayed gratification. Although enjoyable and rewarding academically, medical schools tend to value students with obsessive, self-directed, and nurturing, caring, or somewhat dependent qualities, as these are necessary for most physicians to be successful. On the downside, though, the same qualities make physicians more vulnerable to depression and substance abuse. In addition, 55% of medical students are now female, and for them the delay in having families, or the stress of doing so during medical school or residency, can be extremely significant.

- *Middle adulthood.* Physicians are finally becoming established in their highly valued and respected roles that they have worked toward for many years. Yet they still have to work long and often irregular hours, typically 50–60 hours per week, and most are on call on nights and weekends. So the respect and salaries come with a significant cost to individuals and families, especially the children of hardworking physicians, who may see their parent much less than children of nonphysician parents. For many physicians, there is still lingering debt. In the case of a physician couple in their thirties who are starting a family, and when one of the spouses wants to be a stay-at-home parent for a few years, the combined debt often exceeds $300,000. The consequence is yet more delayed gratification and the deferral of age-usual activities such as joining sports teams, being involved in the community, or attending children's activities. If physicians are going to die by suicide, it is usually toward the end of this phase of their life.

- *Old age.* Physicians are well known to often be resistant to the concept of retirement and confrontation with their own mortality and vulnerability. They often continue working at least part-time well into their 70s, with some continuing much longer. On the one hand, this may be very positive. The intellectual activity is known to be good for the brain, and the skills and experience of senior physicians, whether they are doing volunteer or paid educational or clinical work, are highly valued. The negative side concerns those physicians who literally cannot retire because they have nothing else in their lives. Their whole personality and reason for living is tied up in their professional persona, and some become literally unable to sustain relationships or friendships unless they are in their professional role. Even more important is the obvious fact that physicians are physically human, whatever some might like to believe. From the age of 65 onward the prevalence of dementia doubles every 5 years, so that by age 85 years 25%–50% of seniors will exhibit at least some signs of this disease. The question for older physicians, which will be discussed in detail in Chapter 7, is how they can ensure that they continue to be safe to practice and are not in the early stages of cognitive impairment, which can be very difficult to detect.

This brief developmental summary demonstrates how physicians react differently depending on their age and situation, but it also reveals a number of themes that are common among physicians and that may make it hard for them to seek out help when they need it. Broadly, these relate to physicians' personal characteristics, to community views and cultural expectations of physicians, and to particular medicolegal fears that concern them.

First, as is clear from the foregoing description, physicians need considerable energy, self-motivation, independence, ambition, and focus to be successful and to enable them to overcome the barriers they face and accept the constant delayed gratification through their lives. Thus, they are used to solving their own problems, rather than asking for help, just as Julia was. Asking for help from a colleague is difficult at best—for example, many physicians do not even have their own primary care physician—but is especially so when there is a potentially stigmatized psychiatric disorder, which many see as particularly embarrassing and problematic. So, as is well known, physicians tend to try to treat themselves, and often their friends, family, and colleagues, rather than seek out proper medical and psychiatric assessments themselves. The consequence of this is that physicians frequently receive bad medical care along the lines of the old truism from Sir William Osler: "A physician who treats himself has a fool for a patient." In terms of psychiatric disorders and treatment, the reality is that most nonpsychiatrists know relatively little about psychiatric illnesses. Most received only 2–3 months in total of psychiatric training during their medical school and nonpsychiatric residencies, and for many that was decades ago, and in a field that has changed dramatically in the past 30 years, with a complete transformation of both biological and psychological approaches to treatment having occurred.

The stigma of psychiatry is another major reason for the difficulty in reaching out, and several studies have shown that physicians themselves see psychiatry as being especially stigmatized, and psychiatrists among other physicians even more so. Several major recent studies have examined this issue and have concluded that the internal stigmatization of everything relating to psychiatry by other physicians is related to other physicians' ignorance of the discipline and their lack of understanding of the role of psychiatry, combined with the relatively poor image that psychiatry has had in the past, as exemplified by asylums and coercive treatments. This, of course, is significantly related to the historical separation of much of the practice of psychiatry from other areas of medicine, both geographically and administratively. The consequence is that having to go to see a psychiatrist for treatment is seen by a proportion of physicians, perhaps more so than the general public, as being essentially a personal or moral failure, rather than the need to have treatment from a professional. If psychiatry as a discipline, and psychiatrists themselves, are stigmatized, what does the literature show about psychiatric patients? Here there is even more stigma, with multiple studies showing these patients to be highly stigmatized. It is perhaps not surprising that stigma toward mental illness generally is high among physicians, because this reflects community attitudes where national policies, even today, still do not enable payment for psychiatric disorders at the same rates, or in the same manner, as for physical illnesses.

In this scenario Tom faced another stigma-related problem of significance as a physician, that of his likely being gay, yet feeling he needed to hide this "in the closet" from his colleagues, including Julia, his roommate. Mansh et al. (2015) have described how medical students commonly concealed their identity as "sexual and gender minority" students because they felt it was "nobody's business," through fear of discrimination in medical school or because of social and cultural norms. There are few papers on the experience of lesbian, gay, bisexual, and transgender (LGBT) physicians in the workplace, although a fairly substantial literature exists on LGBT patients showing that living with the stress of disclosure is associated with higher rates of depression, anxiety disorders, suicide attempts, and substance abuse. Eliason et al. (2011) have summarized the literature on LGBT physicians' experiences in the workplace and concluded that, even given the sparse number of studies available, there is research suggesting that medical school and medical practice settings may be discriminatory or hostile work environments for some LGBT health professionals. In their study of 427 LGBT physicians, noting that rates of discriminatory behavior were less than in earlier studies, they still found that 15% of their physician group reported having been harassed by a colleague, 22% had been socially ostracized, 65% had heard derogatory comments about LGBT individuals, and 27% had witnessed discriminatory treatment of an LGBT coworker. While there is no obvious suggestion of discrimination against Tom in the scenario, the fact that he hid his sexual preference suggests that this may have been one of the stressors in his life that contributed to his drug abuse and eventual death.

Finally, many physicians have medicolegal fears and concerns, often unjustified but significant, about being treated for mental health problems. These issues will surface throughout this book. In brief, all physicians have to complete large numbers of forms to gain their medical licenses and to be able to be credentialed to practice in any hospital or health system, and such forms frequently need to be completed every 2–3 years. Almost all of them include one or more questions about the physician's mental health, and many ask about charges of DUI (driving under the influence) or addiction issues, or whether the physician has ever been certified under a mental health act or had their medical privileges withdrawn. So while physicians generally have levels of psychiatric disorders that are similar to those in the age-matched population, they do have a separate concern about their ability and safety to practice and about where the bar is that aligns with this safety level, because that is when medical boards, who regulate physician licenses, become involved. Not surprisingly a potential fear of being reported to a medical board is something that stops many physicians from seeking help. This reluctance to seek help has tragic implications because for the great majority of physicians with psychiatric disorders there should never be any thought of reporting them, since most physicians with psychiatric disorders are fit to practice completely normally. This is another issue, like stigma, where much more physician education is required. It is also an issue that any psychiatrist who is treating another doctor should routinely discuss with the patient so that the physician patient may be reassured that the bar for reporting is actually high, and not low, and relates only to the physician patient's level of clinical competence and the safety of his or her patients and his or her own safety. Having treated hundreds of physicians, I've seen only a handful who would ever consider treating a patient if they knew they were in an impaired state, because on the whole physicians tend to be very conservative when it comes to patient safety, and all are trained to put patients first and to "first cause no harm."

What these concerns mean, of course, is that it can be difficult to convince some physicians who need treatment to accept a referral to a psychiatrist or a mental health professional, just as it frequently is for nonphysician patients. With the advent of the Internet and apps, and an increasing focus on technology in medicine that has enabled more "patient-focused" or "self-care" approaches, there have been more opportunities for creating innovative referral styles, and this difficulty is being overcome. Most people need to be confident that there is a good reason to expend their time and energy to go and see a specialist in any medical discipline. In the field of psychiatry it has only relatively recently been possible to have patients easily and anonymously complete screening questionnaires as in this case scenario. In the past such instruments always had to be handed out and physically completed, and then handed back and scored, so anonymity was very difficult to achieve.

This case demonstrates exactly the process of anonymous self-assessment that the American Foundation for Suicide Prevention has piloted and driven in recent years and that is being implemented in increasing numbers of health systems around the country. This is an effort to engage doctors in treatment ideally at an early stage of their psychiatric illness, well before there is any suggestion of their practice being impaired. The introductory email and the response styles quoted in Julia's case are examples based on actual models used at the University of California, Davis, physician well-being program (http://www.ucdmc.ucdavis.edu/medstaff-wellbeing/), which were modified from originals developed by the American Foundation for Suicide Prevention (http://www.afsp.org/). The UC Davis program has been in place for 4 years (Haskins et al. 2016) and is modeled on a similar program at the University of California, San Diego (Moutier et al. 2012). The survey tool itself is a 35-item online assessment of depression, stress, suicidal ideation, and substance use that uses well-validated questions that are automatically scored and placed in three risk strata for depression and suicide (high, medium, and low). The software incorporates a conversational feature to allow interaction between the monitoring clinical staff and the anonymous individuals completing the survey that can, only if the individuals wish, let them break their anonymity in order to negotiate a referral or an assessment for themselves. This has led each year to about 15 physicians from the 1,800 medical staff at UC Davis referring themselves to psychiatrists or a range of therapists via this tool, in just the same way as happened with Julia. Urgent assessments of medical staff are performed, approximately twice per year, by internal psychiatrists who back up the psychologists who initially respond to emails because the physician's self-assessment suggested significant suicidality. The individuals referring themselves were obviously prepared to trust the system and break their anonymity in a crisis situation. This depression self-assessment tool is now a routine part of the self-care options offered to all UC Davis physicians, residents, and medical students and is an example of the sort of useful evidence-based interventions that are being developed to assist physicians with their health and to reduce the number of physician suicides.

References

Ballard ED, Pao M, Horowitz L, et al: Aftermath of suicide in the hospital: institutional response. Psychosomatics 49(6):461–469, 2008 19122122

Eliason MJ, Dibble SL, Robertson PA: Lesbian, gay, bisexual and transgender physicians' experiences in the workplace. Journal of Homosexuality 58(10):1355–1371, 2011

Haskins J, Carson JG, Chang CH, et al: The suicide prevention, depression awareness, and clinical engagement program for faculty and residents at the University of California, Davis Health System. Acad Psychiatry 40(1):23–29, 2016 26063680

Mansh M, White W, Gee-Tong L, et al: Sexual and gender minority identity disclosure during undergraduate medical education: "in the closet" in medical school. Acad Med 90(5):634–644, 2015

Moutier C, Norcross W, Jong P, et al: The suicide prevention and depression awareness program at the University of California, San Diego School of Medicine. Acad Med 87(3):320–326, 2012 22373625

Scott SD, Hirschinger LE, Cox KR, et al: The natural history of recovery for the healthcare provider "second victim" after adverse patient events. Qual Saf Health Care 18(5):325–330, 2009 19812092

University of Missouri Health Care; forYOU Team: Caring for caregivers. 2018. Available at: https://www.muhealth.org/about-us/quality-care-patient-safety/office-of-clinical-effectiveness/foryou. Accessed January 26, 2018.

Recovery
One Day at a Time

THE NATIONAL ADDICTION annual conference was being held in a large metropolitan hotel as usual. As the speakers for the opening session settled themselves in their places behind the podium on the stage, they looked out at the audience of more than 3,000 taking their seats in front of them. There was an excited bustle of noise, rich with anticipation, filling the theater as the final few hundred registrants entered and searched out the remaining seats. When the seats filled, many had to stand in the aisles at the back and sides of the room.

The lights went down, the audience hushed, and introductory music played as the conference chairman, Dr. Harvey Chase, walked onto the stage. The audience greeted him with a warm round of applause. He took the podium and surveyed the room, taking his time, clearly an experienced and confident speaker.

"Welcome to our annual conference. Yet again we are being well looked after in New York. I look forward to speaking with many of you throughout the next several days, and I do hope you enjoy our national addiction conference, the thirtieth successive event we have held, and with over 5,000 people registered, our largest yet. I want to thank the organizing committee chaired by the current vice president of our Association, Dr. Sandra Podia, for the amazing job that they have performed putting together such an excellent program, which I am sure will prove to be of great interest to you all. The committee has picked, as the theme for the conference, 'solutions and recovery,' and I am sure that our first speaker, who is the embodiment of this theme, will launch our exploration of this theme over the next four days in his own unique style."

Dr. Chase paused, looked around the room as if to try to feel and touch the anticipation of the audience, so eagerly awaiting this opening speaker, and continued.

"We will move straight on to the opening keynote presentation, which I know you are very excited to hear. Let me introduce you to Dr. Andrew MacArthur, who is well known to many. He has spent the past 20 years as a member of Congress representing the great state of Virginia and has been a passionate advocate for the underprivileged, the mentally ill, and those with addictions He has been responsible for numerous legislative initiatives that have markedly improved the lives of hundreds of thousands of people, perhaps millions. Prior to his life in politics Dr. MacArthur was trained as a physician in Boston and, following his residency, practiced in his home state of Virginia as a board-certified internal medicine physician. He is now widely recognized as a beloved national icon and is currently one of the most respected politicians, by both parties, in the country."

Dr. Chase looked around at Dr. MacArthur, seated behind him on stage, looking calm and collected, and wondered what was going through his mind. How could he keep so apparently cool when he was about to take what could well be the biggest risk of his political career, and his life? He sat there, legs crossed, wearing an immaculate dark pinstripe suit, perfectly pressed white shirt, and royal blue silk tie, tall and distinguished looking, with short gray hair in his usual military-style buzz cut. He gazed casually, looking out toward the audience, aware that many had their eyes on him, yet not seeming to be overtly anxious or worried. He looked like he might be about to address a small group in his local constituency rather than a major national convention with a huge press contingent present, all waiting to hear if what it had been rumored he was about to say would actually be said. He appeared a confident man at peace with himself.

Dr. Chase turned back toward the conference, deciding it was time for Dr. MacArthur to take over the podium. "It is my great pleasure to introduce Dr. Andrew MacArthur to all of you. As is customary Dr. MacArthur will speak for about 30 minutes and then we will have time for questions from you, the audience, which, as you all know, you need to submit to me via the conference app so that I can ask them for you. Please do welcome Dr. Andrew MacArthur."

Dr. MacArthur walked to the podium, shaking Dr. Chase's hand firmly as they passed, took up his position behind the translucent glass podium, and waited for the audience's applause to slowly die down. He looked down on the conference attendees, powerfully drawing their attention to him. He seemed to be able to look into the eyes of every individual present, so that even before he began to speak his charisma and self-assurance were obvious and felt by all.

"Thank you, Dr. Chase, and thanks to all of you for attending this important conference. I also wish to thank the organizing committee and the association for inviting me here to speak.

"I am here as a physician who has not practiced medicine for over 20 years, and who has spent most of that time trying to make good the mistakes I made in my life before I went into politics. I have thought long and hard about what I am about to say today and have consulted with many people, especially my family, including my wife of 15 years, Elizabeth, and my two surviving sons, Edward and Hugh. I have also spoken to my political colleagues and mentors and have had tremendous support for my decision to reveal what I am going to tell you today. I know that this will make national news, but I am confident that national attitudes have changed and that I will be understood better now than would have been the case 20 years ago. I am going to tell you the story of my life, in a way that has never been reported previously, and which I have always hidden up until now. I hope to show you that it is possible to overcome the cruelest adversities and tragedies and, for someone like myself, who hit rock bottom in his life, to recover and reclaim one's pride and place in society."

By now the audience was completely still and totally silent. Enthralled by what they were hearing and trying to guess what was coming next. Uncertain. Wondering what his story would reveal. Would the rumors surrounding the tragic car crash in which his wife and son had been killed be confirmed as true? And if so, which of the many differing stories would prove to be correct? Either way the audience sensed it was on the edge of a revelation that would rapidly hit the national media.

Dr. MacArthur looked directly at the audience as he took a deep breath and continued. "They say that the definition of an alcoholic is someone who drinks more than his doctor. Well, in my case that is only partly true because I am both an alcoholic and a doctor." The statement hit the audience forcefully and led to some gasps of surprise. What a sensational revelation from an esteemed national political figure.

"I have chosen today to reveal my disease to you, at this important addiction conference, not only because I am confident you will be a sympathetic audience, but also because I want to show that it is possible to recover fully from the effects of the illness and lead what I believe has been a good and useful productive life, even while continuing the battle for sobriety every day by single day. Do please note that I say that I am an alcoholic now because even though I have over 20 years of sobriety, I know that anytime or any day I could relapse. In my view it is never possible to say that I 'was' an alcoholic because this is a lifelong disorder, one that needs lifelong treatment. So now that you know the secret I have hidden for the whole of my political career, let me tell you more of my story."

On the screen behind Dr. MacArthur a picture appeared. A badly mangled black Mercedes lying on its side in a ditch. Close by, an old, dirty, sand-colored Ford truck, looking battered and worn, was stopped a few yards away from the Mercedes and at an angle that suggested the car had bounced off it before going into the ditch. A series of yellow police tapes ran around the perimeter of the scene, while several official-looking men in suits and uniforms stood near a stationary ambulance on the left of the screen.

"This is in some ways the fulcrum of my story," Dr. MacArthur continued. "It is where my life was changed through tragedy. I have never thought of this dreadful car crash as an accident, because it was so avoidable. Before the crash I was an alcoholic in denial who had constantly failed to take recovery seriously. That was the first half of my life. After the crash I was able, with the support of many people, to gradually recover and gain the confidence to remake my life. So my life really is a story of two very different careers separated by one horrendous event. The circumstances surrounding the smash have, up until now, been hidden from the public record, but I feel it is time to tell what really happened. I hope that others can learn from my mistakes or, more importantly, might be able to gain from them and enter the recovery phase of their alcoholism in the same way as I have done."

Dr. MacArthur walked to one side of the stage, looked up at the wrecked vehicles, and pointed with a penlight to the Mercedes. "Here you see the car that was driven by my wife, Rosemary, and which also contained me in the back, and my son Jake in the front. It has been widely reported that the driver of the truck that hit us was drunk, and at the coroner's enquiry, as many of you will know, he was jailed for 10 years for manslaughter, for the killing of my wife and son sitting in the front seat of the Mercedes as he plowed into our car driving at 60 miles per hour while continuing to drink whiskey from a bottle he kept in his glove box. That is all well known, and the killing of my wife and son by a drunk driver has been widely assumed to be the primary driver of my career change—the reason for me going into politics, and for focusing on the need to create better addiction and mental health services, while giving up my prior medical practice completely. That is of course partly true, but there is more to the story."

Dr. MacArthur paused and then walked to the other side of the stage as if to accentuate the change in direction of his talk. He spoke once more, in a quieter, almost conspiratorial voice. "We went to great trouble to keep the details of the accident as private as possible. It was not easy, especially with my anger and guilt at what had happened, but I hired the best lawyers possible, and they kept the whole process remarkably private."

Dr. MacArthur looked quizzically at the audience. "Why was I not just angry but also overcome with guilt, with shame, with regret? Why did I try and kill myself by overdosing 2 days after the crash, after my wife and son had been killed by a drunk driver? Why did I feel so devastated that I was certified and admitted to a psychiatric unit following the overdose, and kept there for several weeks against my will, missing the funeral for reasons that were explained at the time as 'injuries caused in the car smash'? In retrospect the excuse was fairly accurate, except that the press assumed I had some physical injuries, not psychiatric. Well, to know why I had such an extreme range of emotions, such depths of misery, you need to know more about the circumstances surrounding the crash itself." Dr. MacArthur stopped talking and looked thoughtful, making a decision on where to go next with his story.

"Let me return to the crash later, and why I managed to change my life. I want to tell you a few things about my earlier life and how I ended up an alcoholic. I was brought up in a middle-class home where money wasn't short, but love was. One of my first memories is being told by my dad to clean up my mother's vomit on the kitchen floor. Most of my childhood she seemed to be stuck watching TV in her bedroom, occasionally coming out to shout at us or to look for another bottle. My father kept the house stocked with bottles of vodka and seemed in total denial of her behavior—it was as if he wanted to keep her plastered. He was a successful businessman who worked hard and ignored my mom and his three children. When he had colleagues or other family around to the house, Mom would be literally locked away in her room to prevent her coming out and making a public disgrace of herself. I remember asking my dad about her when I was about 8. He just explained that everyone in her family was like that—her parents and her brother—and that this was just how she was, and we had to look after her because no one else would. She died when I was 14. Drowned in her own vomit and found the next day. None of us cried, and I think my dad may have been relieved. As far as I know she never had any treatment for her disease. She literally drank herself to death over two decades, and Dad kept her situation a secret as much as possible throughout."

Pacing around the stage more confidently, Dr. MacArthur continued. "I was academically bright and hid in my books. So much better than having to think about a dysfunctional home, and a family full of alcoholics, which I now know made me both genetically and behaviorally vulnerable to going down their same path. I started drinking early myself, in my teens, and soon discovered a taste for all sorts of drinks, so that by the time I was in medical school, I was already a regular heavy drinker. I was one of those angry drunks. Most unpleasant to be with when I was inebriated and always wanting to fight, which led to me being arrested twice and having to sleep off my hangover in the local jail. Fortunately, Dad was friendly with the sheriff, so each time I just got a severe talking-to, rather than any charges that might have prevented me from becoming a physician. Medical school for me was a place I swam through in an alcoholic haze much of the time, with a group of heavy-drinking friends and a culture that encouraged us to celebrate or drown our sorrows, always in the same way, in the bar, where I ended up working, which of course just gave me access to lots of free drinks. I managed to keep out of trouble during medical school, and I must have spent some time away from the bar, because I got through and even won a prestigious internal medicine residency position. By now I had been drinking in binges heavily for over a decade, with remarkably good luck, and relatively few associated problems except for a lot of regular headaches and an inability to keep girlfriends, who I always seemed to offend when I was drunk."

He stopped pacing in the center of the stage and seemed to calm down. "In my first year of residency I met Rosemary. We fell in love, and because of her, during the first year of our relationship, I markedly reduced my drinking. We married and had three children over the next 5 years, by which time I was out of residency, and back to drinking, very heavily now but very secretly, so that not even Rosemary knew what was happening. I used to carry a plain blue water bottle with me everywhere and no one noticed it. Of course, I didn't have water in the bottle, but straight vodka, which I was continuously drinking throughout the day. All day every day. I became like my mother, a compulsive drinker. I kept myself topped up all the time and was able to hide my intoxication well, I thought. Finally, one of the nurses picked up on my behavior and started to see that I would be irritable after several hours of being scrubbed up for my endoscopy list but suddenly calm down and act differently an hour after the end of the list following a trip to the change rooms. Anyway, this nurse took a sip from my water bottle one day when I had left it in the change room and immediately realized it was vodka, not water. She reported what she had found to the chief of gastroenterology, who called me into his room and confronted me. Now, this was before the existence of good treatment programs or a true understanding of the disease of alcoholism. My chief was a friend, and while he was angry and disappointed by what had been found, he decided not to punish me if I agreed that he could tell my wife so that she could help me, and if I promised not to drink on duty again. After all, from his perspective, this was my first time drinking on duty, because I lied about what I had been drinking, and I was happy to promise him whatever he wanted. Remember, this was almost 30 years ago. A very different time and approach to what would have happened to me now, and an ineffectual action completely lacking in consequences. As is well known I have been promoting controversial legislation to make random drug and alcohol testing required for all physicians, and now you know the reason for it. If it had been in place when I was practicing, my alcoholism would likely have been discovered earlier."

On stage Dr. MacArthur was more reflective, with the audience entranced and at the same time fascinated by his story. "To cut a long story short, I was soon back drinking heavily again, although now Rosemary knew about it. The next 5 years consisted of me constantly trying to stop drinking; failing; going into detox several times and rehab twice; seeing all sorts of therapists, psychiatrists, addiction counselors; and taking Antabuse and various antidepressants. Whatever potential treatment was the flavor of the month, I tried it. Rosemary constantly supported me and, in retrospect, probably enabled me by being too supportive and forgiving. We managed to keep my drinking fairly secret as my career went on a downhill path. I moved out of the academic medical center to private practice, where there were fewer people to observe what I was doing, so I managed to keep drinking heavily and quietly, working most of the time and often quietly intoxicated, until the car crash. That's when my life finally changed for the better, although it was too late for Rosemary and Jake.

"Let me move on to the second half of my life, and treatment. What I have learned is what works and what does not. What has helped me and what has been ineffective. As I mentioned, I was severely depressed and suicidal for months after the crash and ended up spending over 4 months in the hospital, for combined treatment of depression and alcohol dependence. I was fortunate in being treated by a strict no-nonsense psychiatrist who did not give me any special favors because I was a physician, unlike most of the other doctors who had treated me previously. In comparison to them, whom I was able to fool for years, he made sure I was carefully followed up and constantly monitored. He was used to treating alcoholic physicians, so he knew all the tricks of their trade. Doctors such as myself are frequently considered by many treating doctors to be VIPs, and it is now well known that such VIPs tend to get poor treatment because they are intimidating. Fortunately, my psychiatrist was not at all intimidated by me and immediately arranged for me to have 3 months in an alcohol rehab facility where there was a specialist program for professionals whose work was dependent on them being licensed to practice. People like doctors, lawyers, and pilots. Here I completed the first eight steps of the Alcoholics Anonymous 12-step program and then followed this up as an outpatient, where I continued daily meetings, as I still do today. I have found that it is so important to go to meetings with people that you can relate to. In the early days I used to go to what we called "caduceus meetings"—that is, meetings for health professionals—and after moving into politics and beginning to spend most of my time in Washington, I started attending meetings with other politicians, staffers, and aides. I was shocked to find how many alcoholics are working on the Hill successfully as public figures. Many of us sponsor other colleagues who are alcoholics, especially those who are new to Congress. I know that I have partially transferred my addictive tendency from drinking to compulsive daily attendance at groups, so that when I am traveling, the first meeting that goes on my schedule each day is the time and place of the local AA group.

"I have thought a lot about my treatment. I still see a psychiatrist once per month regularly, as someone who knows me well and can oversee and monitor my treatment, because I will never fully trust myself to do this because I know how easily I can deceive myself. I have had a lot of psychotherapy over the years, mainly focused on my losses and the damage I have done to myself and others through my drinking, and have still not fully worked through all of these issues, which is perhaps partly why I am baring all today to you. I have been treated with several different medications. I took antidepressants for several years after the crash and was on high doses during the year or more that my suicidal ideas persisted. For many years I was on Antabuse, a drug to make me feel sick if I drank, and for the last 10 years, I have taken naltrexone to reduce the cravings for alcohol that I still sometimes have. I think that the therapy and medications are key components of what has helped."

Dr. MacArthur had been speaking as if he was giving a lecture, but now he quieted and moved to the front of the stage, almost as if taking the audience into his confidence.

"All of these treatment approaches are fairly conventional, but I still have a daily challenge not to drink, so I have two other very specific and constant external daily controls that I find really helpful and that I wish other alcoholics would use. My psychiatrist says that he uses these fairly routinely now with most of the alcoholic physicians whom he treats. First, I have an app on my phone that I complete every single day and that sends my answers to my wife, Elizabeth, so she can know how I am feeling, wherever I am. On the app I have to specifically tell her I have not had a drink that day. I could never lie to her after what happened to Rosemary, so she is what I think of as my loving daily truth monitor. My second external truth monitor is proving that I am alcohol free, not just telling people that I am clean, so I voluntarily undergo routine random breath analysis, with the results sent to my psychiatrist. In the old days, having body fluid analysis like this meant going to have several urine tests per month at a lab, which was very inconvenient. Now I do all my monitoring by telemedicine. I log in to a Web site every morning and randomly, four times per month, the Web site requires me to send in a breath sample within 8 hours of logging in. I carry a digital alcometer with me wherever I go, literally in my shaving kit. This has a camera attached to the alcohol monitor so that whenever I breathe into the monitor, the camera takes a picture of me, to show there is no cheating; time-stamps the digital photo; adds the breath analysis result; and sends the completed visual data direct to my psychiatrist, to my alcohol app, and to my wife. I find this voluntary external monitoring incredibly useful in keeping me honest and on the correct pathway in life.

"And talking of telemedicine, that is how I usually see my psychiatrist now. It is simply more convenient for both of us, as we both have busy lives, and since I always have a laptop or iPad with me. It is good to see him in person occasionally when I am back at home, but most of the year when I am mainly in Washington, I just log in to his video room for my regular monthly appointment and see him from wherever I am. I have been seeing him like this for almost a decade now, and it has made such a difference to my life. I used to worry about having to go to his clinic in case I was recognized in the waiting room, but now I have much more privacy seeing him on secure video from my home or office, so telemedicine treatment has been really positive for me. I have referred a number of other colleagues from Congress to him, and he has told me that he has found it very interesting professionally to have what is now a congressional telemedicine practice. He usually sees me from his home, which is apparently what happens with most of his other video patients, so the whole process seems to be a win-win for all of us."

Dr. MacArthur took a deep breath and waited silently on the center of the stage. An isolated figure picked out by a spotlight. The audience sensed another revelation. "So I have managed to combine a comprehensive treatment program for my lifelong disease with a life in politics. I do hope that the approach I have taken—one that combines therapy, AA and group programs, sponsoring others, medications, and external monitoring—is a helpful example that others might follow. Yet I have done one other thing that not all people need to do, or would want to do. I have totally changed my career and my life. I stopped practicing medicine. I went into politics. And of course, thankfully, I found Elizabeth and have made a wonderful life with her. Not everyone goes to these extremes, so why did I do this?"

At the flick of his finger Dr. MacArthur brought back the slide of the car smash and turned around toward the dreadful scene. For the first time he seemed to be anxious and worried, clearly reaching the most difficult part of his story. "Think about the Mercedes. Why was I in the back, at 11 in the morning? The answer is simple. I was dead drunk and fast asleep. I cannot remember a thing about the crash itself. My long-suffering wife and son were driving me home after yet another 3-day bender during which I drank continuously, out of contact with them, until I either ran out of money or literally fell down in the street and got picked up yet again by the police. In this instance both things had happened, and my wife and son had just driven 50 miles to find me and take me home. So it is true that I changed the direction of my life as a result of the crash caused by a drunk driver, but what was not known until now is that there were two drunks that caused the deaths of my wife and son. If I had not gone on that bender and had to be 'rescued,' my dear wife Rosemary and my son Jake would likely still be alive. They would not have been driving me home and would not have given up their lives for me."

Dr. MacArthur looked visibly distressed as his voice broke. He turned back to the screen, where a happy family photo appeared. "Here they are," he said shakily. "This was taken a month before Rosemary and Jake died. There they are—Rosemary obviously next to me, and Jake in between his two younger brothers, always the one to look after them, until the disease of alcoholism killed him through no fault of his own. The irony of the crash was that it was caused by two alcoholics, one drunk driver and one incapacitated passenger, and they were the only two who survived." Dr. MacArthur stopped talking and let the family photo have an impact on the audience. A few people could be heard sniffing. The room was now full of emotion. Dr. MacArthur standing quietly, alone, on the right of the stage, suddenly looking a smaller and more tragic figure, no longer the confident man who had previously dominated the room. Now uncertainly trying to judge the reaction to his revelation.

"So you can see why I was suicidal. Racked with guilt. Ashamed and afraid to speak to anyone. Just wanting to give up and die. Alcoholics don't just harm themselves. This is a family pursuit, and all are involved. Up until then I had not realized how much potential harm I could do to others when I went on a bender. It took me a long time to decide to move forward with my life. I decided that I just could not trust myself to ever work as a physician again. After all, I had learned how to practice while intoxicated for years, and I had no idea how much harm I had done, how many people I had treated less well than should have been possible. Whether I had made any serious mistakes. Anyway, I was reported to the medical board after the crash by the coroner as part of a deal that my lawyer managed to make when my past history came out. It soon became obvious that the best I could hope for from them was a probationary license and that I would be lucky to get that. I spent a lot of time in therapy with my psychiatrist at the time going into the various options I had. In the end, after he had to write a report for the medical board, in which he very honestly said that he thought my prognosis as an alcoholic was poor and that I was unlikely to maintain long-term sobriety, I voluntarily surrendered my medical license. This was a few months after the crash, and after I was out of rehab and sober. So that explains why I stopped practicing medicine and why, instead, I went into politics. Well, believe it or not, there were three reasons initially."

Dr. MacArthur stopped to sip from a glass of water placed near the podium and turned back to address the audience, now close to the end of his story, and his speech full of stunning revelations.

"As I have mentioned, I had always been interested in politics and was well connected politically. Well, one of the interesting things about being a member of AA is that you meet the most interesting people from all walks of life at AA meetings. In my case I met a state senator, who I will not name, who eventually became my AA sponsor, and lifelong mentor, and he encouraged and supported me along this path. Second, I was bored and depressed. I had nothing to fill the gap left by giving up my medical practice and the death of my wife and son, although as a single dad of two surviving young boys I did have a lot of parenting to do. I found being involved in politics gave me an interest again, and so I gradually got more and more involved and connected, and a year after the crash, with the retirement of my local congressman, I took a risk and campaigned for the first time in my life. Third, and this came up in therapy a lot, I saw politics as being potentially therapeutic for me, for two reasons. The obvious one that is in my public bio is that I wanted to help others with mental health and addiction problems, and that is absolutely true, and I am proud of my legislative successes over the years. The less obvious reason, though, is something that my psychiatrist has allowed me to see. In politics I am a public figure. If I relapse and have to be rehospitalized or admitted to detox, it will be completely public and totally humiliating. It will be another reminder of my failure with Rosemary and Jake and of how I was at least partly responsible for their deaths. It will be a public letdown of my very supportive wife, Elizabeth. It will be shameful. So going into politics has in effect been part of my therapy. It is something that has ensured that I remain sober and do good, rather than being able to cover over my drinking as I could as a physician, when I quietly left academia and went into unmonitored private practice."

Dr. MacArthur returned to the podium and looked at the audience. "I want to finish by thanking all of you for listening to my personal story. Hopefully there are some nuggets in there that may be helpful to some of you. For me it has been a difficult decision after over 20 years to finally be honest with the world and to tell my complete story. I know I am going to be criticized by some, and I deserve it for all the years that my behavior put my patients at risk. I hope that you, as health professionals who work in the area, will not let people like the man I was 20 years ago, like maybe one of your colleagues, go untreated. Physicians with this disease need you to help them acknowledge the disease so they can begin the process of treatment and healing. Ignoring alcoholism in physicians is a dangerous path for everyone concerned. I know that I have also caused much suffering, but I am committed to being healthy and a productive person. Now I am ready to take a few questions. Thank you for listening."

Commentary

This case raises several important issues regarding the common problem of physicians with alcohol abuse and dependence, which are also addressed in Chapters 1 and 6 in particular. First, the case demonstrates the importance of implementing evidence-based treatments for alcohol dependence in physicians, and not allowing them to receive second-best care because of their potential VIP "special patient" status. Second, this case highlights extra factors that need to be taken into account to successfully treat physicians who have alcohol (or drug) disorders, especially those involving voluntary or involuntary random body-fluid monitoring and screening in the workplace, as well as the need for medication-assisted treatment and professionally relevant individual and group therapy programs. Finally, this case illustrates how technology is revolutionizing medical care, and how technology and digital devices, monitoring apps, and telemedicine can be used with physicians to monitor the course of their illness over many years and to maintain confidential therapeutic relationships with their providers, while also involving their families as necessary.

Much has been written about the many and varied assessment and treatment approaches used with patients who have alcohol-related disorders, so the details will not be included in this book, except as relevant to treating physicians as patients. An excellent recent guide by Levounis et al. (2016) covers the literature in a comprehensive and thorough manner, discussing the epidemiology and neurobiology of addiction and current assessment and treatment approaches for alcohol use disorder (AUD), including alcohol dependence. They note the common co-occurrence of psychiatric disorders, especially depressive, anxiety, and posttraumatic stress disorders, with medical comorbidities, especially gastrointestinal, cardiovascular, and neurological disorders. They report that the lifetime prevalence of AUD is 30% and that alcohol is involved in about 40% of motor vehicle accidents in the United States. The National Institute on Alcohol Abuse and Alcoholism (2017) reports incidence rates of 6.2% among adults over 18 (8.4% among men, and 5.3% among women) for AUD, with more than 1.3 million adults receiving treatment at a specialized facility in 2015 and an average of 88,000 people dying from alcohol-related causes annually, and another approximately 10,000 dying through alcohol-impaired driving fatalities (representing 31% of all motor vehicle deaths per year).

The importance of these numbers in relation to physician health is that there is strong evidence to show that physicians have at least as high rates of AUD, which includes alcohol dependence, as age-matched control subjects in the general population. Figure 4–1 shows a comparison of diagnostic criteria for AUD from DSM-IV (separate conditions for alcohol abuse and dependence) and DSM-5 (alcohol use disorder includes alcohol dependence), with DSM-5 defining the severity of AUD as mild (2–3 symptoms), moderate (4–5 symptoms), or severe (6 or more symptoms).

The treatment of individuals with AUD is still varied and at times controversial, entailing a number of differing philosophical and, therefore, practical approaches. The main core issue is differing views on whether patients should attempt to gain complete sobriety with total abstinence, or whether it is reasonable, in some individuals, to attempt "controlled drinking" aimed at harm minimization or harm reduction outcomes rather than total sobriety outcomes.

	DSM-IV — In the past year, have you:	#	DSM-5 — In the past year, have you:	
Any 1 = ALCOHOL ABUSE	Found that drinking—or being sick from drinking—often interfered with taking care of your home or family? Or caused job troubles? Or school problems?	1	Had times when you ended up drinking more, or longer, than you intended?	The presence of at least 2 of these symptoms indicates an **Alcohol Use Disorder (AUD)**. The severity of the AUD is defined as:
	More than once gotten into situations while or after drinking that increased your chances of getting hurt (such as driving, swimming, using machinery, walking in a dangerous area, or having unsafe sex)?	2	More than once wanted to cut down or stop drinking, or tried to, but couldn't?	**Severe:** the presence of 6 or more symptoms
	More than once gotten arrested, been held at a police station, or had other legal problems because of your drinking? ****This is not included in DSM-5****	3	Spent a lot of time drinking? Or being sick or getting over other after-effects?	**Moderate:** the presence of 4 to 5 symptoms
	Continued to drink even though it was causing trouble with your family or friends?	4	Wanted a drink so badly you couldn't think of anything else? ****This is new to DSM-5****	**Mild:** the presence of 2 to 3 symptoms
Any 3 = ALCOHOL DEPENDENCE	Had to drink much more than once did to get the effect you want? Or found that your usual number of drinks had much less effect than before?	5	Found that drinking—or being sick from drinking—often interfered with taking care of your home or family? Or caused job troubles? Or school problems?	
	Found that when the effects of alcohol were wearing off, you had withdrawal symptoms, such as trouble sleeping, shakiness, restlessness, nausea, sweating, a racing heart, or a seizure? Or sensed things that were not there?	6	Continued to drink even though it was causing trouble with your family or friends?	
	Had times you ended up drinking more, or longer, than you intended?	7	Given up or cut back on activities that were important or interesting to you, or gave you pleasure, in order to drink?	
	More than once wanted to cut down or stop drinking, or tried to, but couldn't?	8	More than once gotten into situations while or after drinking that increased your chances of getting hurt (such as driving, swimming, using machinery, walking in a dangerous area, or having unsafe sex)?	
	Spent a lot of time drinking? Or being sick or getting over other after-effects?	9	Continued to drink even though it was making you feel depressed or anxious or adding to another health problem? Or after having had a memory blackout?	
	Given up or cut back on activities that were important or interesting to you, or gave you pleasure, in order to drink?	10	Had to drink much more than once did to get the effect you want? Or found that your usual number of drinks had much less effect than before?	
	Continued to drink even though it was making you feel depressed or anxious or adding to another health problem? Or after having had a memory blackout?	11	Found that when the effects of alcohol were wearing off, you had withdrawal symptoms, such as trouble sleeping, shakiness, restlessness, nausea, sweating, a racing heart, or a seizure? Or sensed things that were not there?	

FIGURE 4–1.   Comparison of criteria for alcohol use disorder between DSM-IV and DSM-5.

Source.   National Institute on Alcohol Abuse and Alcoholism (https://pubs.niaaa.nih.gov/publications/dsmfactsheet/dsmfact.htm).

Alcoholics Anonymous and related 12-step-style programs histori-cally aim for abstinence as the primary outcome, but studies have shown that 60%–90% of individuals who enter 12-step programs drop out or fail to maintain abstinence, often as a result of the insistence on withdrawal and the "cold turkey" approach to care. This has led to the increasing pop-ularity of motivational interviewing, in which the positive and negative sides of sustaining the negative behaviors are emphasized, leading the in-dividual to make up his or her mind as to how quickly and how much to proceed with the harm reduction approach. This is often done with the help of counseling, either individual or in a group, with a focus on individual em-powerment and choice, which is very different philosophically from the AA abstinence approach.

The choice of whether patients should try for abstinence or might con-tinue drinking moderately depends on the patient's clinical factors and personal preferences. Patients who are compulsive drinkers, who cannot have one drink without then moving on to finish a whole bottle, and who cannot keep alcohol in their house as it will be too much of a temptation to finish it should generally be advised to try for abstinence. Others who are less compulsive may be advised to keep to the maximum recommended level of 10 drinks per week for males, or 8 for females, keeping a diary of use for monitoring purposes, and asked to keep at least 3 days per week alcohol free so that they do not drink constantly and become physiologi-cally dependent. These individuals are practicing harm reduction by reducing their total alcohol intake and avoiding adverse physical complications, as well as reducing their capacity and likelihood to have major binges.

A secondary, increasingly less controversial issue is the place of medi-cation-assisted treatment, which in the United States has tended to be un-derused for many years because of the prevalence of abstinence programs, but which is now gaining in popularity as the evidence supporting this ap-proach increases. The first and most obvious approach is to use medica-tions to treat any concurrent psychiatric illnesses that individuals with AUD have quite commonly. Such disorders include depressive disorders, anxiety disorders, bipolar disorder, posttraumatic stress disorder, and ob-sessive-compulsive disorder; and for each, specific combinations of anti-depressants, mood stabilizers, and tranquilizers are available. The second approach is to use medications specifically for the alcohol problem itself. These are well covered in Levounis et al. (2016), and only brief details will be included here. Two of these drugs, naltrexone and acamprosate, reduce the craving for alcohol that many patients have and that scientists have been trying to understand for many years. These investigations assume that there is a "craving gene" whose expression can be turned on and off by certain medications, hence making drinking less likely. Naltrexone is available orally and can be taken each day, but it is also available by injection, whereas acamprosate is only available by injection. Both drugs, when taken regularly, are associated with markedly less drinking overall in patients. The third drug, and the oldest, is disulfiram, commonly known by its trade name, Antabuse, which is taken orally. If the patient taking this drug ingests alcohol, the toxic metabolite of alcohol builds up in his or her body, the breakdown of the metabolite being inhibited by disulfiram, and results in very unpleasant symptoms, such as flushing, sweats, nausea, and vomiting. In many patients this "disulfiram reaction" is enough to stop them from drinking. The downside, of course, is that it is easy for patients to stop the drugs that they take orally and wait a couple of days before they then get back to drinking.

Physicians who enter carefully monitored treatment programs for alcohol or substance abuse that focus on complete sobriety, with or without medication-assisted treatment, do extremely well, and long-term studies report that about 75%–90% of them are actively practicing and have retained their medical licenses at 5 years, which is a very much better outcome than the prognosis for most age-matched nonphysicians (Yellowlees et al. 2014). Some variations among specialties have been noted. Anesthesiologists, for example, not surprisingly suffer disproportionately from opioid dependence because of their easy access to narcotics, rather than alcohol dependence, and surgeons appear to have a lower rate of return to clinical practice, although their 5-year successful completion rate is comparable to that of physicians as a whole. Family physicians successfully complete the 5-year programs less commonly, however (Rose et al. 2017). Psychiatrists, in a study by Yellowlees et al. (2014) examining the outcomes of 55 psychiatrists, showed no differences for these doctors from the overall cohort of 904 physicians, despite the stigma surrounding this profession and the stereotype that they are more vulnerable to substance use disorders and mental illness.

It's highly likely that Dr. MacArthur's drinking patterns met the DSM-5 criteria for severe AUD in the latter part of his years in medical practice, but while he was at medical school, he probably had mild AUD. It is remarkable to think that approximately 6% of the current practicing group of physicians in the United States meet at least two of these DSM-5 criteria. We know that the natural unchecked progression of alcohol abuse over time in many people, especially for those with genetic vulnerability, is for gradual progression through to alcohol tolerance and dependence, as per items 9–11 in the DSM-5 criteria, and that physicians are extremely adept at hiding their use. This seems a strong argument for the introduction of random drug and alcohol testing for all physicians to both prevent physicians from going down the path from mild to severe disorder, and especially to pick up those individuals who are binge drinking or for whatever reason practicing in an intoxicated state with alcohol in their system at work.

Levy (2017), in her review of the issue of random drug testing of physicians, reported that in a survey performed by Medscape in 2016, 41% of 7,500 physicians said doctors should be tested for drugs. She further noted that the practice of random testing of employees is growing in acceptance. She quoted one physician who pointed out that military medicine has been doing random drug testing of all healthcare workers since the 1980s, and that as long as there is a robust chain-of-evidence security process, such an approach seemed very reasonable, while other physicians supported the need to detect physicians who might eventually die by suicide as a result of overdose. While there are always going to be those who oppose such a move, the rationale for implementing random drug and alcohol testing of physicians seems strong, and such testing should be implemented to improve physician health, as well as to protect patients and enhance patient safety. The example in this chapter, where Dr. MacArthur was able to practice unmonitored and unchecked, regularly intoxicated at work, for several years, is unfortunately not uncommon, and it is impossible to tell what poor decisions were made on patients during that period of time. Without doubt there are many patient errors made by such intoxicated physicians, and these need to be reduced.

Dr. MacArthur went through many years of failed treatments for AUD prior to the fatal car crash and commented that he was pleased, after his suicidal thoughts, to no longer be treated as a VIP patient by his new psychiatrist. VIP patients can be any persons who are unusually influential, such as physicians, celebrities, the politically powerful, or the very rich, who in association with their behavior can influence their treating physicians' behavior or judgment. Alfandre et al. (2016) have reviewed the process of caring for VIPs and have examined the ethical dilemmas that this raises and made suggestions for the improved practical management of such patients, as discussed further in Chapter 8. These authors note that while this identification may improve rapport, it can also blur clinical objectivity and may lead to poor clinical reasoning and decision making. The ethical values in conflict here are those of autonomy of the patient versus beneficence (promoting the best interests of the patient), in which the role confusion may lead to a change in care.

Another ethical issue of importance for physician VIPs relates to privacy. Physicians are often public figures, and having them sit in a waiting room, where they might be recognized by other staff from the same health institution, or may even be next to some of their own patients, is clearly a problem. There are many instances of reporters trying to access health information on celebrities, which is what Dr. MacArthur certainly became during his political life. Sometimes extra services need to be provided to protect certain individuals' privacy, and this can be ethically justified, as Alfandre et al. (2016) note, because of the ethical need to be able to treat all patients in an equivalent manner.

For a number of reasons, including privacy and the wish to be treated in a professionally understanding environment, as well as the importance of achieving sobriety for certain licensed professionals such as pilots, physicians, and lawyers, as well as other health professionals, a number of inpatient and outpatient programs have been developed specifically focused on these groups. It is straightforward to find such programs in many states via Internet search engines using search terms such as "addiction treatment for health care professionals." They tend to focus on specific workplace challenges, such as easy access to, and knowledge about, drugs, irregular work hours, and the impact of repeated emotional traumas experienced at work, as well as all the other more generic issues involved in treatment. A number of them also specifically examine the personality strengths that are important in health professionals, such as caring (or dependency issues), perfectionism (compulsive anxiety), and problem solving (time pressures), and how these can also become risk factors for addiction. These programs often also work with employers, who may have insisted a health care employee attend, perhaps via a physician well-being committee, as discussed in Chapter 9. As such, they may well offer a return-to-work assessment, including recommendations on fitness to practice and detailed recommendations for follow-up clinical care, perhaps in conjunction with a recommended network of providers, as well have the capacity to write reports as indicated for licensing boards, monitoring programs, employers, or any other professional groups involved with the individual.

In the case described in this chapter, it seems that Dr. MacArthur's long-term psychiatrist was respectful of his patient's training as a physician but at the same time was prepared to insist that Dr. MacArthur stay in the hospital and obtain appropriate treatment (under legal order) for his depression and suicidality, and then his AUD, just as the psychiatrist would have for any other patient. In later years the psychiatrist started using telemedicine to treat Dr. MacArthur, and this was an ethically appropriate improvement in his care because the use of telemedicine to his home was likely to be more protective of his personal privacy than making him attend an outpatient clinic.

The final issue of importance for discussion in this chapter is the use of clinical health technologies, such as telemedicine, to care for patients. There is strong evidence that their use can lead not only to better access but to a higher standard of care and a more flexible and consistent doctor-patient relationship for physicians with psychiatric or addiction-related problems than is possible with purely traditional in-person approaches to care.

Over his many years of treatment, Dr. MacArthur became a regular user of telemedicine for his clinical consultations and also used apps and his alcometer for self-monitoring and for communicating his data with his treating doctor and, in his case, his wife. *Telemedicine* has been defined broadly by the American Telemedicine Association (2018) as "the remote delivery of health care services and clinical information using telecommunications technology. This includes a wide array of clinical services using internet, wireless, satellite and telephone media." Historically, telemedicine has included a variety of modalities to deliver care, such as video-conferencing, telephone, email, Internet and apps, fax, and still imaging, both synchronous, in real time, and asynchronous, or store and forward, in delayed time, and is now encompassing virtual reality, big data environments, and algorithmic processes and workflows with data analytics and predictive assessments on the fly. In short, telemedicine is generally thought to include all information technologies, even mobile apps, designed to be used at the patient-provider interface.

Bashshur et al. (2015) completed the most recent review of the evidence concerning the feasibility, acceptance, cost, quality of care, and health outcomes of telemedicine interventions in mental health. This review, which studied children, adults, the elderly, veterans, and different ethnic groups, in both urban and rural settings, found that while telemedicine certainly improves access to mental health care, it also enables providers to effectively deliver a range of psychotherapies as well as improves the efficiency, quality, and cost-effectiveness of care. The other recent review (Hilty et al. 2013) of the effectiveness of telemental health compared with in-person care found that telemental services are effective for diagnosis and assessment across many populations, for many disorders and in many settings, including when integrated in primary care, and are comparable to in-person care. Hilty et al. (2013) concluded that such technologies are now good enough to allow patients to be treated in their homes or communities, rather than requiring them to travel to places such as hospitals and clinics.

Several authors have described how the future standard of multimodal clinical care for patients with psychiatric and addiction disorders will likely be hybrid care with telemedicine and mobile technologies being integrated into primary care systems (Chan et al. 2015; Yellowlees et al. 2015), and with patients being seen in person and online, depending on mutual convenience, in much the same way as described in this case. A recent systematic review of Web-based tools and mobile applications to mitigate burnout, depression, and suicidality among healthcare students and health professionals by Pospos et al. (2018) featured seven programs designed to enhance breathing, meditation, or suicide prevention, as well as providing Web-based cognitive-behavioral therapy. The development of handheld alcometers that are accurate and photograph the users as they test their breath is a large step forward in addiction management in that it allows accurate body fluid monitoring and reporting anytime anywhere, and in a way that is much cheaper and more convenient than insisting that a patient visit a laboratory. Equally, the many apps available to measure mood levels, report questionnaire responses, and share data with agreed recipients significantly increase the potential for self and external monitoring of individuals with alcohol and substance disorders (Yellowlees and Shore 2018).

References

Alfandre D, Clever S, Farber NJ, et al: Caring for "very important patients"—ethical dilemmas and suggestions for practical management. Am J Med 129(2):143–147, 2016 26522793

American Psychiatric Association: Diagnostic and Statistical Manual of Mental Disorders, 5th Edition. Arlington, VA, American Psychiatric Association, 2013

American Telemedicine Association: What is telemedicine? 2018. Available at: http://www.americantelemed.org/main/about/about-telemedicine/telemedicine-faqs. Accessed January 26, 2018.

Bashshur RL, Shannon GW, Bashshur N, et al: The empirical evidence for telemedicine interventions in mental disorders. Telemed J E Health 22(2):87–113, 2015 26624248

Chan S, Parish M, Yellowlees P: Telepsychiatry today. Curr Psychiatry Rep 17(11):89, 2015 26384338

Hilty DM, Ferrer DC, Parish MB, et al: The effectiveness of telemental health: a 2013 review. Telemed J E Health 19(6):444–454, 2013 23697504

Levounis P, Zerbo E, Aggarwal R: Pocket Guide to Addiction Assessment and Treatment. Arlington, VA, American Psychiatric Association Publishing, 2016

Levy S: Is random drug testing in physicians' future? July 11, 2017. Available at: https://www.medscape.com/viewarticle/882399. Accessed January 26, 2018.

National Institute on Alcohol Abuse and Alcoholism: Alcohol use disorder: a comparison between DSM-IV and DSM-5. 2017. Available at: https://pubs.niaaa.nih.gov/publications/dsmfactsheet/dsmfact.htm. Accessed July 2017.

Pospos S, Young IT, Downs N, et al: Web-based tools and mobile applications to mitigate burnout, depression and suicidality among healthcare students and professionals: a systematic review. Acad Psychiatry 42(1):109–120, 2018

Rose JS, Campbell MD, Yellowlees P, et al: Family medicine physicians with substance use disorder: a 5-year outcome study. J Addict Med 11(2):93–97, 2017 28067757

Yellowlees P, Shore J (eds): Telepsychiatry and Health Technologies: A Guide for Mental Health Professionals. Arlington, VA, American Psychiatric Association Publishing, 2018

Yellowlees PM, Campbell MD, Rose JS, et al: Psychiatrists with substance use disorders: positive treatment outcomes from physician health programs. Psychiatr Serv 65(12):1492–1495, 2014 25270988

Yellowlees P, Richard Chan S, Burke Parish M: The hybrid doctor-patient relationship in the age of technology—telepsychiatry consultations and the use of virtual space. Int Rev Psychiatry 27(6):476–489, 2015 26493089

The Conundrum of Treating the Physician Addict

THE LARGE COMMUNITY CENTER was packed, mainly with elderly people, but also with a number of younger severely disabled individuals sitting in wheelchairs at the front. An unusually high proportion of the audience members were wearing or holding a variety of medical supports and devices—neck braces, slings, and walking canes. They were all intently listening to the professionally dressed woman center stage who appeared to be powerful and somewhat domineering while at the same time convincing as she spoke.

Dr. Colleen Ward paused; surveyed the hundred or so people in front of her, trying to make as much eye contact with them as she could; smiled; and looked down briefly at her last PowerPoint, showing her professional contact details at the rheumatology clinic she had founded, including her phone and email address. She waited to make sure she had everyone's attention and then continued on to finish her talk.

"I hope you've enjoyed this presentation. Let me finish by briefly summarizing what we've discussed. I've focused primarily on the management of chronic pain. As you all know, this is common in people who have chronic arthritis and musculoskeletal disorders. We know that narcotic painkillers, and similar potentially addictive substances, are highly effective for most people with acute pain, and that as long as patients are properly screened before such medications are prescribed, only a small number of people will become addicted when these medications are used for long-term treatment. In my own practice, with our careful procedures, I believe this is a rare occurrence, and we find that our multidisciplinary approaches, combining medications and a variety of procedures and therapies, are highly effective in most patients. We are very aware of the concern that patients have about the possibility of opiate addiction, but it is important to remember that 75% of narcotic addicts start their addiction careers as young people using a number of illegal and prescription drugs. We also know that most people, when they start taking narcotics, take drugs that have not been prescribed for them. In other words, they take drugs that have been diverted from their original prescribed purpose, whether they were prescribed for a family member or acquaintance, or were bought or otherwise obtained on the streets. In most studies, only 10%–15% of people addicted to opiates started their addiction as a result of pain treatment from a doctor. So the message to all of you who have chronic pain is to work closely with your doctors to obtain the best pain management regimen that you can, and use that in combination with all the other lifestyle and meditation-related changes we have discussed tonight. If you are taking any form of narcotics, all of which are potentially addictive, do make sure that no one has access to them, especially your children. Keep them locked up and either return all unused medications to your pharmacy or destroy them so that they cannot be stolen or used by others. Chronic pain is a dreadful condition to have, but with the right individually customized treatment, I assure you that most patients do very well and can get back to highly functional lives. Now, I know we have a few minutes to spare, so I'm happy to take any questions that you have."

Dr. Ward remained standing, listening to the enthusiastic applause from the audience, and anxiously watched for the raised hands of those with questions. This was often the most difficult part of the evening from her perspective. Almost always some patients asked her about their own treatment, and she wanted to be very careful not to publicly criticize any regimens being ordered by other physicians, however odd they sometimes seemed to be. She was only too aware that prescribing medicine was both an art and a science and that however many guidelines and formal treatment recommendations from professional bodies existed, every patient was an individual. She knew that some patients seemed to do better on unusual combinations of medications that might look odd on first inspection but that might have been arrived at through a careful process of trial and error. As usual, on this evening the questions were a combination of personalized treatment queries that were difficult to answer and questions expressing concern about the addiction potential of some of the painkillers, especially narcotics, and how this could be minimized or avoided. She answered all the questions in her usual competent and thoughtful manner, listening carefully to the concerns behind all the questions, but at the same time trying to always answer using theoretical responses, and outlining principles rather than getting into specific individual clinical details. Partway through the Q&A session her phone started buzzing repetitively. She glanced down, trying to be unobtrusive in front of the crowd, and saw a series of texts from her latest partner, Janet, who was demanding her attention urgently. She decided to finish the questions as rapidly as she could and sent a brief text to Janet telling her she would be home in 15 minutes.

Janet rushed to the door when she heard the car in the drive. She was at least 10 years younger than Colleen and was wearing a pink tracksuit and worn gold slippers, with her auburn hair up, tied casually in a bun at the back of her head. She looked tired, with dark circles under her puffy eyes, and was clearly agitated and immediately demanding of Colleen, speaking in a whining childlike voice. "Why do you have to go out and give these talks? I want you to be home more—I hate having to text you, to almost beg you to come home. This is such a nice place to be. We need more time together now that we're an item. I've been all strung out waiting for you so long. Did you get the narcos I asked for?"

Colleen responded in an irritated voice. "Yes, Jan, of course I have the Oxys that you asked for. You know I'm never going to let us run out of those. How do you think I would manage without them? You should have had enough with what I left here for you this morning. Did you take them all earlier today? How many times do I have to tell you that you should take them more regularly, not a lot at one time, then you can still feel good and not have any withdrawals, and at the same time not run out? How do you think I get through my average day seeing patients? I need to take the narcos regularly and make sure I don't appear to be intoxicated by taking too many. It's actually quite straightforward once you get used to it. And it's really important that you take them better because I know you think I can get unlimited supplies, but it's hard, and I have to be very careful so that no one gets suspicious, especially the pharmacists. They are all completely paranoid about opiates and the potential for drug addiction nowadays and check everything so carefully. And what's more, with you here, I now need to get a lot more than I used to get when it was only me who needed them, so it's sometimes harder for me."

Colleen stopped and took a pill bottle out of her coat pocket and proudly showed it to Janet, who by now had settled on the couch in front of her, pouting and acting childish and spoiled in response to Colleen's lecture. "Here you are."

Janet grabbed at the bottle and expertly took the childproof lid off, not looking at the label or checking the contents. She took four tablets out and almost seemed to inhale them. She threw the pills rapidly into her mouth, followed by a large gulp of white wine.

Colleen sat down opposite her and continued talking. "Luckily I saw a new elderly patient today who has a lot of pain from her bone cancer and who needed to start on regular narcos. As usual I suggested that, as a favor, I could pick up all her new meds for her on my way home and drop them off at her home. She was blown away that her doctor is so caring that she will do that, because it's hard for her to get out much now. Anyway, that gave me the opportunity to have the pharmacist give her a large supply, which I dropped off at her home earlier on. I was able to take about a third of her pills for us, and she was just so pleased to see me that she didn't notice the bottle wasn't full. She's a really nice lady. She even introduced me to her two beautiful show dogs and asked if I might be interested in going to a dog show sometime with her. I'm sure she'll never miss the pills, and if she's OK with me continuing to pick them up every time she needs some more, we'll get a good, regular supply from her, even if I end up needing to go to one of her dog shows. Hopefully this will last for many months until she has to go into hospice care, at which point the nurses will take over her medications and I won't be able to divert her pills for us."

A few days later at work Colleen was busy as usual. She was a very popular doctor who worked in her solo practice with several nurses and physician assistants as well as a therapist, in a clinic she had designed herself. For a rheumatologist, she had a large patient panel, especially of patients with chronic pain in association with their various musculoskeletal disorders. She knew that many of her patients came to see her because she was prepared to treat them with long-term narcotics, as had been her practice for many years, but others came because she had a reputation as being a very patient-centered physician, who always went the extra mile to help them. She knew that she sometimes became over-involved in her patients' lives, and her mentors over the years had often talked to her about her difficulties with boundaries in her relationships with patients and in her personal life. She preferred to think of herself as someone who was very giving and concerned and who always tried to help others who had more needs than she had. So when the phone rang and her receptionist was busy on the other line, she picked up the handset to answer the call herself, expecting to have a patient on the line who would be grateful at being able to speak directly to her. She could not have been more wrong.

"Could I speak to Dr. Colleen Ward, please?"

"Certainly, this is she."

"Dr. Ward, my name is Gerard Lock, and I am an investigator from the medical board. We have had several reports concerning your prescribing practices recently and I would like to come and discuss them confidentially with you. Are you available at 5 P.M. tonight for me to come to your clinic?"

Colleen was suddenly flustered and worried about what could have been reported. She replied anxiously, "Well, yes, I suppose so. I'm usually finished with patients by then, so I have time. Can you tell me more about what this is about?"

"I am sorry, it is better if we talk about it in person. Just so you know, I will have a colleague with me and we will be recording our interview as part of the investigation. I look forward to meeting with you tonight. Thank you for being available."

At that, Mr. Lock ended the call, leaving Colleen suddenly worried and fearful about what had been reported. She had always been concerned that a pharmacist would discover what she was doing. She had been taking her patients' narcotics for a number of years and using them herself, and sometimes giving them to friends like Janet. Most of the time she had done this by taking some of the drugs she had prescribed for her patients, but she had also written many prescriptions for several family members that she had picked up supposedly on their behalf at different pharmacies. As a doctor with a narcotic addiction, it was all so easy to get her own supplies. She had discovered that there were relatively few checks in the system to stop a prescriber from obtaining controlled substances like narcotics for themselves. As long as she varied the individuals she took drugs from, she felt safe, especially since she wrote a lot of completely genuine prescriptions for narcotics for her patients with chronic pain and was known as an expert in that area. She had long ago overcome the guilt about using drugs that were meant for her patients, some with cancer pain, and who consequently went without their whole supply and likely had to tolerate more pain than necessary. Colleen knew that she herself was a narcotic addict, but she felt that as long as she was careful and did not increase the doses of her drugs and kept herself fully able to function both socially and at work, she would be fine. She rationalized her use of narcotics as good overall, as they allowed her to remain healthy enough to look after her many patients. She no longer had the awful mood swings, sometimes so severe that she was suicidal, that she had had in the past as a medical student and resident, when she had used all sorts of substances like alcohol, marijuana, meth, and cocaine to try to make herself feel better. She thought of her use of large doses of narcotics in recent years as being almost the equivalent of self-medicating to calm herself and cope with the difficulties she had always had with relationships. She had deluded herself into thinking she could maintain her habit permanently.

She spent the rest of the day in an anxious, distracted mood, although she did not forget to take the four OxyContin tablets she needed to take at noon and 4 P.M. as usual.

Eventually 5 P.M. came and the pair of investigators from the medical board were seated in her office, recorder on. They explained that no accusations were being made but that they were there to obtain a statement from her in the expectation that it would explain the complaint they were investigating.

Mr. Lock, who was apparently the senior investigator, started the discussion.

"We have had three separate reports from local pharmacists about some of your patients. In all three cases the pharmacists were concerned that some of their patients' narcotics had gone missing, as they seemed to have received fewer tablets than prescribed by you. In all cases you had volunteered to take the medications personally to their homes, and all of these families had later gone back to the pharmacy to try and obtain more pills when the patients' supply as given to them by you had run out. We do not know what happened but wonder if you have any explanation as to how they could have run out so soon."

"Can you tell me the names of the patients so I can check my notes? Obviously some patients are more reliable than others, and it's possible that they could have lost some of their medications, or even taken too many, especially if they were the sort of individuals who might get confused sometimes," Dr. Ward responded confidently. "I'm happy to look up their notes and give you some more information about them."

"That would be most kind," Mr. Lock continued. "We will do that in a few minutes. At the same time I would like to make copies of all of your notes for those patients so that we can have an expert that we employ also review them."

Dr. Ward was affronted by this suggestion, reacting irritably. "Why do you need to get someone else to review these confidential medical notes? Surely you'll accept my word on what I think happened?"

Mr. Lock looked up from his papers and hesitated before replying. "Well, normally we would not need to get such a second opinion, but you see, there are some other concerns that we have about your prescribing practices, and so we feel we need to be very thorough and careful to make sure we have all the correct information."

"It really does seem that you don't believe me. What's going on?"

"Well, you see, the problem is that we have done some extra checking around, and we do feel the need to double check all that has been happening. It is in your interests and ours that we are very careful and do a proper investigation of these complaints. You may not be aware of this, but you are one of the highest prescribers of narcotics in the whole state. We have checked your prescribing records and have already had them broadly reviewed by an expert in pain management, who tells us that it is hard to understand why you need to prescribe so many patients such high doses of narcotics. This especially applies to some patients who seem to have terminal cancer, like the three patients who we want to review with you."

Mr. Lock continued talking. "As part of the investigation we have gone through the state narcotics database and have made a complete list of all the individuals for whom you have prescribed narcotics in the past 6 months. We want to compare this list with the patients you have registered in this practice, because one of the pharmacists, in her report to us, told us she had been surprised by two young women who had presented prescriptions for OxyContin written on your prescription pads, and who she thought might be addicts. So you can see that there are several issues we need to discuss and review."

Throughout this discussion Mr. Lock remained friendly and nonjudgmental so that despite his suspicions, he would appear to be as objective as possible. He had interviewed a lot of doctors over the years and had found that the great majority were honest and reasonable, with nothing to hide, but that they were human, like everyone else, and sometimes made mistakes, or practiced in an unusual way, although with the best of intentions. He wanted to make it clear to Dr. Ward that he really did want her opinion on some odd circumstances and cases and that he was quite prepared to believe her version of events if it made sense.

Dr. Ward, however, was having none of this. She had managed to hold herself together while Mr. Lock spoke, but she now reacted very defensively and angrily. Such outbursts used to be common and had occurred many times in her life, whenever she felt challenged or threatened. This time she was driven on by the confidence emanating from the large dose of narcotics she had taken just an hour before.

She pulled herself up in her chair, as if to try to dominate the conversation and the room, and spoke with passion and annoyance, unable to hide her contempt and anger at being challenged.

"Well, this is certainly not what I was expecting. I don't know what you really want. I planned on being fully cooperative with you, but I don't like what I am hearing. It sounds like you have had some very minor complaints against me where it seems that these people are trying to label me as a drug addict, or inappropriate prescriber, or whatever. You know pharmacists are always keen to overrule a doctor. I'm just a very hard-working doctor who happens to be an expert in chronic pain and who therefore prescribes a lot of controlled substances. Of course I prescribe more than most other doctors. I am a rheumatologist, and most of my patients are in pain. Some busybody pharmacists have had the nerve to report me when the most likely explanation is that the patients lost their meds. We all know that they do that all the time, especially if they are on narcotics that can make them a bit confused sometimes, so they may take too many pills and not remember. And as to how my prescriptions were obtained by possible addicts, if that's what they were, I have no idea what was going on, but there is a simple explanation for that, if they were not my patients. One of my prescription pads must have been stolen. That does happen, you know. Or do you people always just assume the doctor is the problem and then come to harass us? It's not that uncommon for doctors to have their pads stolen by light-fingered patients, however closely we watch them."

Dr. Ward seemed to run out of steam, flustered by the underlying accusations, and her anxiety at what was going on. She took a deep breath, settled back further in her chair, calmed herself, and continued talking, more slowly now, and in an affronted but wary manner. Less overtly hostile and wanting to give herself more time to think.

"This is all just a witch hunt. You are trying to access my confidential medical records and compare them with your state databases, which in themselves may be wrong. Have you thought of that? You're trying to prove that I'm doing something wrong when I'm just doing my job. I feel really insulted and have never been treated like this in my life. I don't want to continue this conversation and think you should leave. I have no intention of breaking the confidentiality of my patients' records by giving you access to their charts and intend to consult my lawyer as to what is the best approach to handle your awful, insulting insinuations."

Mr. Lock and his female colleague sat and listened in surprise at this extraordinary outburst from a doctor who they had heard had an excellent reputation. While it was true that they were investigating the pharmacists' complaints and were naturally suspicious due to the nature of their work and training, they did not really expect to find anything major at fault where Dr. Ward was concerned. But this outburst, and her angry refusal to cooperate with them, raised a lot of red flags. As Mr. Lock stood up to leave, he said, "Dr. Ward, it is your prerogative not to cooperate with what we believe is a straightforward investigation. I need to warn you that your lack of cooperation will be seen as a serious issue, and we will need to consult with our colleagues and legal advisers at the medical board. We will be back in contact with you after that so that we may progress with this investigation."

The next week was a nightmare for Colleen. She was constantly afraid that Mr. Lock, or another of the medical board investigators, would appear at her clinic. She knew that they would be coming back to her soon and that the consequences would likely be serious. She was rational enough to know that her addiction was going to be found out and that her life would be changing dramatically soon. She was afraid that they might stop her from practicing, but she had little idea of any other potential consequences or actions they might take. She was perpetually on edge and checked her mail anxiously, looking for documents from the medical board. Whenever the phone rang, she jumped internally but no longer picked up to answer herself, always leaving that for one of her staff. She even took to carefully making sure all the people in her waiting room were really her patients, in case one of them might be there incognito to serve her some legal papers on behalf of the board.

She continued working, however, and, as she had many times in the past, she tried once again to reduce the number of OxyContin pills she took each day. She told herself she would be able to taper off them herself and tried yet again to convince herself that she was not really physically dependent on narcotics. Her withdrawal symptoms of irritability, moodiness, agitation, and anxiety, combined with muscle aches, insomnia, sweating, yawning, and a runny nose, gradually increased, forcing her to confront a different reality—one where it was obvious to her that she was a narcotic addict in withdrawal. She finally had to confront this truth. All of this made it increasingly hard for her to concentrate on her work or her patients' needs, and she became increasingly agitated, especially at home with Janet, who she could see was really only staying with her in order to have a regular supply of drugs. Her relationship with Janet had deteriorated, with one fight after another over the past several weeks. Finally, she asked Janet to leave following several serious arguments that started when she said she could no longer be her drug supplier. Janet took off for good, leaving Colleen feeling deserted and used but somewhat relieved.

After a few weeks Colleen had managed to cut the number of pills that she was taking each day in half, but she was a wreck and found that she was starting to crave alcohol, or almost any other drug, to help cover her narcotic withdrawal. She had no appetite and was losing weight. She couldn't sleep and was feeling exhausted, defensive, and paranoid. At that point she decided she had to seek some advice. She couldn't do this alone, but she had failed so many times in the past, why would she succeed now? She had no idea how to find someone to talk to urgently and confidentially, and certainly had no intention of speaking to any of her colleagues about her circumstances. She realized she had no real friends anymore. She had withdrawn from people over the years as her addiction had taken over her life. How could she admit that she was an addict? What a stigma. What a humiliation. She thought long and hard. She didn't want to go to see her own primary care doctor or use her health insurance for this sort of problem because she didn't want to have her history known to her insurers. She would rather pay cash if she had to, but who could she see? Getting treatment as a physician for an addiction was just too humiliating. She finally decided to phone the state medical association's "physician help line" that was set up as a service to all physicians who were suicidal or had psychiatric or substance-related problems and were in crisis. She knew that she fit this description all too well and decided that she couldn't do herself any harm speaking to one of the volunteer physicians, mostly psychiatrists or addiction-boarded physicians, who were available via this line.

Colleen spoke tentatively into the phone. "Hello. I'm a specialist physician, and I need some help with my addiction. I've tried to withdraw myself, but I can't do it alone. I think I need to go to detox somewhere before I lose my medical license. Can you help me, please?"

The anonymous physician at the other end of the line responded: "I appreciate how hard it has probably been for you to ask for help. I don't need to know your name or any personal details at this stage, but obviously if you decide you want us to arrange some help for you after we have spoken, then I will need to know who you are. You said you have an addiction and you think you need to go to detox. Before we go any further I just want to check that you are feeling safe and are not thinking of hurting or killing yourself, because if that is how you are feeling, we need to discuss that first."

"No. I appreciate you being so direct with me. That's not how I feel at the moment, although I have thought of taking an overdose a few times over the past several years, and I did take one when I was a medical student. I don't feel I'm at risk of doing that just now and have no plans to hurt myself. I do feel very out of control though, and I know that if I don't get some help and change my situation, I could feel like that again." Colleen broke down in tears on the phone, hardly able to talk, distressed and upset. She continued to listen to the sympathetic anonymous voice.

"I am glad that you are not feeling immediately at risk of overdose. Perhaps you could fill me in on what has been happening recently and how you think I can help. Take your time. There is no hurry."

"I'm addicted to narcotics. I've been taking them for years. Mainly OxyContin tablets recently, but all sorts of other narcotics, stimulants, and tranquilizers in the past. I've managed to keep it hidden until recently, but it has just gotten out of control, and now the medical board is investigating me and is bound to find out what is going on. I've managed to keep practicing all the time, but I'm afraid they will take my license away and I'll lose everything. I have been doing some reading online about physicians in my situation and found an article that said that if I could get into treatment voluntarily, and before the medical board took any action against me, I might be able to continue practicing once I am completely off the drugs. I know it's awful to be a doctor who is addicted. I feel so ashamed. I can't tell any of my friends or colleagues, although I suspect some of them will not be completely surprised when they find out, as I guess they will."

"How long has this been going on? Can you tell me some more about what has happened to you?"

Colleen continued, at times speaking rapidly, letting her story flow in a torrent. "A long time. I used cannabis quite a lot in medical school, and like all the students I hung out with, I drank quite heavily most weekends. Then the drinking expanded beyond weekends and was especially heavy after exams were all finished, and with friends when we were partying, especially at the end of our courses or rotations. I was mixing dope and booze until I would pass out. I wasn't much different from all my student friends, especially those in medical school, except that I found it very hard to keep relationships, and I lived a fairly chaotic social life. That wasn't surprising, I guess. I come from a weird family and was orphaned after my parents both died from drug-related problems, and then I had a really difficult time as a teenager in many different foster homes, where all sorts of bad things happened that I probably haven't put behind me. The good news was that I had brains and used to hide in my books as a teenager. Schoolwork was the only place I got any peace and where I felt confident, but I was always moody. I was one of those students who was up and down a lot. I could never be good enough and lacked confidence, although no one would have known that because I learned to cover up my feelings. I guess alcohol and drugs were a defense for me even then. I had lots of boyfriends and also a number of girlfriends as I experimented, often under the influence of alcohol or cannabis. The overdose I mentioned occurred after a relationship breakup and my second abortion. Anyway, I got through medical school and, apart from my difficulty with relationships, think I did much better in residency, which I really enjoyed and where I was just too busy to use many drugs."

By now Colleen was feeling calmer and less worried about this conversation. She liked the sound of the phone counselor and felt confident in him, so she continued.

"When I completed my internal medicine residency and fellowship, I worked in the hospital system for a decade, and have been in private practice the last few years. My use of prescribed drugs really started about a year after I finished my fellowship. I had what I thought was a serious relationship at last, and was very committed to Paul, but he just couldn't stand what he described as the pressure of being in a relationship with a doctor. I earned twice as much as he did, and he just didn't have the confidence to stay with a professional woman. I know so many of my female doctor friends who have had the same problem—there just seem to be few men who can relate comfortably to intelligent, assertive professional women. Anyway, Paul dropped me for no good reason and started going out with a blond bimbo who worked in a retail store. I was devastated and heartbroken. Because I really loved him, but also because I was 10 times the woman he eventually married. So I guess I started using drugs about then. I was given a prescription for some tranquilizers by a fellow doctor to help me sleep initially, and I rapidly increased the dose and was soon writing my own prescriptions in other people's names. It just went on from there. The tranquilizers led to me feeling too tired and dopey during the day, so I added stimulants like Ritalin. I liked the feel they gave me but managed to control them for a while and thought I was managing OK. Then I had to have a minor shoulder operation for an old tennis injury, and the orthopedist gave me a full bottle of OxyContin to take after the day surgery. There were 60 tablets in the bottle, and while I probably only needed 5 or 10 from a clinical viewpoint, having this whole bottle was like Christmas for me. I had never taken any narcotics before that time, but I just loved how they made me feel, and I managed to consume the whole bottle in under 10 days. Then it was a matter of continuing this new habit rather like I had managed the tranquilizers and stimulants, except that I had to be much more cunning writing prescriptions for my patients and for imaginary individuals so that I could keep my supplies going. And believe it or not, I've managed to do that for the past 7 or 8 years, keeping myself going on a regular six to eight tablets per day. Most of the time it has been OK and I've kept everything very carefully secret. I've had two girlfriends, most recently a woman called Janet, who must have almost picked me out, because they both used me as a supplier for themselves and, when I caught on, left me. There goes that relationship issue again. I so wish I was better at them."

Colleen stopped talking and reflected on her situation. Although she had been doing most of the talking, she also had a series of questions she wanted answered. She continued.

"I'm sorry. You probably don't need to know my whole history. I just haven't ever told anyone in this sort of detail before, and it seems a bit odd, even to me, hearing it like this. You wanted to know what has happened recently. Well, the bottom line is that I have been reported by three different pharmacists who have been watching my prescribing patterns, and the medical board is investigating me. I have thought long and hard in the past week about whether I should just admit what has been going on to them, and hope that they will understand, but I really don't know what to do. Should I get a lawyer? I know I'm going to need help to detox, because I can't do it by myself, and I guess that may mean I'll need to go to rehab, as I can't imagine coming off these drugs as an outpatient or while I'm still working. So what do you think I should do? Can you advise me? I have had to accept that I am an addict. I don't like it, and I feel very ashamed. Goodness knows what you think of me. I should be able to do better than this as a doctor. But I do know doctors are at risk of addictions because we can get hold of drugs so easily, so I realize I'm not alone. You've probably spoken to many others like me. How have they done? Is it possible for me to come back to a more normal life, where I am not constantly working out where to get my next prescription from and how to avoid detection? It's all just so tiring and exhausting that I can imagine it may actually be easier to be sober. I have to get some help. I'm so lonely, and my life is such a mess. I can't go on like this. Can you help me?"

Three months later Dr. Ward walked into the spacious office and sat down opposite Dr. Martin, the medical director of the most prestigious drug and alcohol treatment facility in the state. It was her last session with him after her 3-month residential stay, initially for detox, and then medication-assisted therapy, initially with buprenorphine and then naltrexone, as well as rehab and a range of psychotherapies, involving a modified 12-step program with individual and group sessions. She looked and felt like a different person from 3 months previously, smartly dressed with her long blond hair neatly pulled back in a tortoise-shell clip, and having put on some much-needed weight.

Dr. Martin started the conversation. "Well, this is a big day for you. Congratulations on your achievements here. As we've agreed, it's time for you to leave, and I want to review how you've done here and discuss your future treatment plans."

Commentary

Dr. Ward's history of self-prescribing and polysubstance abuse, with eventual narcotic addiction, is fairly typical, especially for female physician addicts, who tend to abuse prescribed drugs, in contrast to their male colleagues, who more commonly abuse alcohol. Dr. Ward appears to have come from a family where she was genetically and behaviorally at increased risk for drug dependency, and most likely suffered a range of physical and/or sexual abuses during her time in foster care. She seems to have always had a rather histrionic and borderline personality style (American Psychiatric Association 2013) characterized by mood swings; difficulties in relationships, especially with social and sexual boundaries; and an angry, defensive and dramatic style of protecting her fragile inner world, especially when handling conflict or threats. Not uncommonly for physicians with drug problems, medical school was a time when her symptoms first emerged, although residency was a time of relative calm for her, when she poured herself into the long hours of work required of her. Dr. Ward also seems to have done reasonably well prior to going into private practice, but once there, with the usual relative lack of professional structure and collegial observation seen in small practice environments, she relapsed and began her drug abuse, in a setting where access for her, as a physician, was relatively easy. Her excessively dependent style of living was demonstrated in her relationships with her patients, where she crossed professional and social boundaries, partly to help her obtain drugs, and in her sexual relationships, where she seemed unable to find rewarding matches and ended up choosing drug-addicted partners, which added greatly to her risk-taking behavior. Fortunately, she is someone with a lot of strengths as well, especially her intelligence, her capacity to keep working, and her ability finally to admit to her problems. She seems to have done well in rehab and in a 12-step program, and it is hoped she'll continue to do well in future with appropriate monitoring in a long-term treatment program.

So what have we learned from Dr. Ward's story?

1. Doctors who have significant medical or psychiatric histories in family members may be at increased genetic or behavioral risk of developing related disorders, but these same family histories and healthcare experiences are commonly a reason for them choosing medicine as a career. Not surprisingly, they suffer from all the same sorts of developmental abuses and difficulties that occur in the general population.
2. Substance abuse is frequently associated with suicidal ideation or suicide attempts.
3. Doctors with substance use disorders frequently do not arrange treatment for themselves, or admit that they have a problem, until many years have passed and their addiction is severe, or its impact is great, or both.
4. Doctors tend to be very resilient and resourceful and can hide substance abuse highly effectively, often for many years, especially if the substance being abused is being obtained at work, as with prescribed drugs.
5. Dr. Ward's substance abuse was severe, with craving and tolerance, such that she was physiologically dependent on narcotics. This was why she constantly failed to manage her own withdrawal successfully. In this setting, the best form of treatment for her long term was likely to be complete abstinence, with a range of psychotherapies, regular monitoring of behavior and body fluids, and medication-assisted treatment as the best combination of evidence-based approaches available. In an individual like Dr. Ward, with a lost career as a likely consequence of relapse, harm minimization approaches, where she would be allowed to take small regulated amounts of some of the substances she abused, such as alcohol, would be less likely to be successful.

Dr. Ward's case brings up a number of important discussion issues around substance use and abuse and the barriers that exist that stop physicians from seeking care. The following are some important basic facts about physician addiction:

• The lifetime rate of addiction among practicing physicians is likely 10%–15%, which is about the same as in the general population overall.
• Alcohol is the most commonly abused drug by physicians, with alcohol use disorder occurring at about the same rate as in the general population.

- Doctors have higher rates of prescription drug abuse (particularly opioids and benzodiazepines) than the general population and tend to use nonprescribed drugs less.
- Untreated substance use significantly increases the likelihood of physician suicide.
- As a result of stigma and the threat to their license and professional reputation, addiction of all types is often advanced by the time physicians seek treatment.
- Although doctors face significant personal and professional challenges, one advantage they have is access to physician health programs, which can lead to excellent outcomes, with more than 80% of physicians drug-free and practicing in their discipline 5 years after referral to these programs.

Physicians, like the general public, use and abuse the full range of prescribed and nonprescribed drugs (Substance Abuse and Mental Health Services Administration 2015), although it is prescribed drugs, such as narcotics and benzodiazepines, which they have better access to, that, after alcohol, are physicians' usual drugs of choice. A recent position paper on this issue from the American College of Physicians by Crowley et al. (2017) confirmed that substance use disorders involving illicit and prescription drugs are a serious public health issue and that in the United States millions of individuals need treatment for substance use disorders but few receive it, which mirrors the situation with physicians. This paper noted that the rising number of drug overdose deaths and the changing legal status of marijuana pose new challenges. Importantly, the American College of Physicians maintains that substance use disorders are treatable chronic medical conditions and offered a series of recommendations on expanding treatment options, especially with medication-assisted treatment, to address the opioid epidemic, as well as education and workforce and public health interventions. (See Chapter 4 for a discussion of alcohol abuse and dependence.)

There have been a number of self-report studies examining the prevalence of physician substance abuse, but accurate estimates are unknown, although presumably the prevalence data mirror national data for nonprescribed drugs. The amount and types of substances used by physicians have changed significantly over time, so that, for instance, in the last 40 years, in the light of our knowledge of the adverse impact of smoking on health, physicians have dramatically reduced smoking. In the last 10 years, however, the increased clinical presence of prescribed drugs, along with the greater number of female physicians in the physician workforce, has meant an increase in the number of physicians who have become dependent on opioids and benzodiazepines. What the changes in marijuana legislation occurring currently, with decriminalization in some states, will do regarding physician health, and the capacity to practice, is uncertain. It's inevitable, however, that increasing numbers of physicians will start using marijuana, and this issue will have to be thought about soon at both national and state levels. It will be interesting to see if many follow the informal policy of the Colorado Physician Health Program, as described by Johnson (2012), whereby any physicians "who legally use medical marijuana to treat their own debilitating conditions such as chronic pain or nausea are considered unsafe to practice medicine in the state of Colorado until such time that they no longer need the treatment."

What we can estimate from the literature reviewed in Chapters 4 and 5 is that of all physicians who have substance use disorders, about 50%–70% use alcohol, 30%–35% use prescribed drugs (usually opioids or benzodiazepines), and the remaining 5%–10% use cocaine, methamphetamine, and marijuana or other hallucinogens.

The next question asked by many is whether some specific medical disciplines carry a higher risk of developing substance use disorders than others. This issue has been fairly extensively researched, even though, because of the secretive nature of the behaviors, this research is hard to do accurately. The best current answer from the studies quoted below is that physicians from emergency medicine and anesthesiology tend to become addicted to narcotics more frequently than physicians from other disciplines, and that females tend to become more frequently addicted to tranquilizers than males (who tend to use alcohol more than females do). All of these findings, which will be discussed in what follows, really relate to access to the drugs rather than to the actual disciplines involved. So what do the studies show?

Hughes et al. (1999) carried out the most extensive physician specialty comparison performed at that time, and nearly 20 years later findings from this study merit repeating, as community drug usage has changed markedly during this time. In this self-report study with a 59% response rate, 5,426 physicians from 12 specialties responded. The researchers found that emergency medicine physicians used more illicit drugs, psychiatrists used more benzodiazepines, and anesthesiologists used more opiates. Pediatricians and surgeons had low use, except for cigarettes, and self-reported substance abuse and dependence generally were highest among emergency physicians and psychiatrists and lowest among surgeons. The other series of studies relevant to this issue have arisen from the work of McLellan et al. (2008), who evaluated the outcomes of 904 physicians with diagnoses of substance abuse or dependence who were consecutively admitted to 16 U.S. state physician health programs. This data set has been reanalyzed several times to examine specific discipline outcomes and prevalence by substance type, and a number of findings are especially relevant here:

1. Emergency medicine physicians had a higher rate of substance disorders, with proportionately more use of opioids, than other physicians but also were more successful in treatment and return to practice (Rose et al. 2014).
2. Anesthesiologists suffered disproportionately from opioid dependence rather than alcohol dependence but had similarly good treatment outcomes to the other physician groups (Skipper et al. 2009).
3. Psychiatrists were not overrepresented, and 5-year outcomes for this discipline were similar to those of other disciplines, although there was a higher proportion of females in psychiatry (Yellowlees et al. 2014).
4. Family medicine physicians had rates of substance use disorders that were similar to those for other physicians, but they were less likely to successfully complete 5-year monitoring contracts (Rose et al. 2017).
5. Surgeons appeared to have a lower rate of return to clinical practice, although their 5-year successful completion rate was comparable to the rates for other disciplines (McLellan et al. 2008).

Why, then, do physicians become drug addicted as Dr. Ward did? There are of course many reasons that are covered throughout this book. All physicians, like members of the general population, are unique and differentially affected and driven by a large range of genetic, biological, psychological, and social pressures, including all the documented risk factors for addiction, especially childhood trauma and the presence of psychiatric disorders. A number of specific physician-related stressors have been identified, all of which affected Dr. Ward:

1. *High educational demands.* American medical students have a history of using alcohol, benzodiazepines, and prescription opiates at a higher rate than their student peers while working long hours with competitive pressures in a culture that endorses substance use as a way to cope with stress.
2. *Patient care.* Providing medical care can be rewarding and difficult. Unexpected outcomes and treating difficult or noncompliant patients are challenging, and until recently few physicians received adequate training to manage these stressful patient care issues.

3. *Long hours.* The feeling of always being available, with long work-days and trips to the hospital at all hours of the day and night, not only is mentally and physically exhausting but interferes with family, recreation, and self-care, such that physicians often end up eating badly, exercising only occasionally, and sleeping poorly.
4. *Availability of addictive substances.* Access to drugs is part of day-to-day practice and always a temptation.
5. *Failure and fear of reporting.* While physicians have a professional duty to report colleagues who may be practicing while impaired, numerous studies suggest that few will actually do so when faced with this situation, or will simply not recognize an impaired colleague. Although physicians may feel that this type of professional courtesy is a good short-term response, it unfortunately enables addictive behaviors and prevents addicted doctors from receiving the help they need. Such a conspiracy of silence is frequently perpetuated by family and friends of the addicted physician.

Given all these data, and the obvious importance of treating physicians with a substance use disorder while at the same time ensuring that they remain fit to practice and patient safety is not compromised, what sorts of treatments and treatment approaches are most appropriate and effective for physicians? This is quite a conundrum. Exploring the evidence base of all treatments for individuals with substance use disorders is beyond the scope of this book. It is possible, however, to broadly summarize the potential range of treatments available for a physician like Dr. Ward. Most physicians choose residential detoxification and rehabilitation, for up to 3 months, at a variety of programs set up around the nation that specifically cater to professionals like physicians, pilots, and lawyers, all of whom have licensing concerns. The next major decision is whether to choose *opioid substitution treatment* (OST) supported by a range of psychotherapies, or *abstinence-based psychosocial treatment* (ABPT). This is not an easy decision, but historically, even though current guidelines support the use of OST, most physicians have chosen ABPT, primarily because the physician health programs that they are likely to be referred to for monitoring in most states have either written or informal policies insisting on physicians' body fluid samples being completely negative as a way of ensuring patient safety.

It is well worthwhile to examine both sides of this issue because there's not a clear conclusion at present. The American Society of Addiction Medicine (ASAM; www.asam.org) defines addiction as "a primary, chronic disease of brain reward, motivation, memory, and related circuitry, with a dysfunction in these circuits being reflected in an individual pathologically pursuing reward and/or relief by substance use and other behaviors" (ASAM 2015). A full review of current evidence-based treatments for individuals with opiate dependence, a chronic relapsing disease, is available from ASAM (2015), and this review strongly supports the implementation of OST. The comprehensive treatment guideline from ASAM covers assessment and treatment options, including treatment for opioid withdrawal and the use of substitution medication-assisted treatment involving methadone, buprenorphine, or naltrexone, as well as the importance of psychosocial treatments used in conjunction with medications. In the guideline ASAM notes that their preferred term "for this serious bio-psycho-social-spiritual illness" is "addiction involving opioid use." There is a lot of evidence to support the use of OST, and that approach to opiate addiction is increasingly becoming the standard of care in the United States. Despite this, there remain several concerns regarding the efficacy of OST that are particularly relevant to those with an interest in physician health. First, nonphysician patients being treated often continue illicit opioid use, and treatment dropout is common, although both could be reduced with careful monitoring in physician health programs. Second, treatment with OST is often recommended for life because of the inherent risks of attempting to taper to zero dose, and the idea of lifelong OST may be incompatible with physicians' licensure restrictions or other regulations.

Despite the guideline recommendations described above, OST was not planned for Dr. Ward because in her state the monitoring program she was going to be involved in, run by the medical board, insisted on complete sobriety and negative random urine screens for opiates. Dr. Ward was being discharged from a rehab program after a 3-month stay, during which she was initially detoxified using tapered doses of methadone and clonidine, as per the ASAM guideline. However, after detoxification she was not given medication-assisted treatment (such as OST) and was treated exclusively using ABPT.

What is the evidence in support of this approach? Merlo et al. (2016) have recently reviewed the various treatment approaches for narcotic addiction that are currently available and used with physician patients. As part of their review, Merlo et al. compared treatment outcomes among substance-dependent physicians enrolled in a long-term physician health program (such as the one Dr. Ward was being referred to) who had a history of alcohol use only, any opioid use, or nonopioid drug use. They found that 75%–80% of physicians across the three groups never tested positive for alcohol or drugs during their extended care management period of up to 5 years with random drug testing. This included physicians with opioid dependence who did not receive OST. The researchers concluded that physicians with opioid use disorders can achieve long-term abstinence from opioids, alcohol, and other drugs through participation in ABPT with extended, intensive care management following discharge.

Intensive ABPT usually consists of residential treatment, which is what Dr. Ward received, or a partial hospitalization program consisting of several hours of therapy several days per week at minimum. Both these options usually comprise a range of individual and group psychotherapies, usually with a cognitive-behavioral conceptual base. There are usually regular process groups to evaluate progress, family therapy with involved spouses and sometimes children, recreational or work-related therapies, educational programs, and often an introduction to a 12-step program that may be continued after the residential treatment is completed.

It seems clear that there is reasonable evidence supporting both sides of this debate, although there is almost no evidence of the efficacy of the use of OST in physicians as a special group of patients, mainly because this treatment approach is seldom tried with them, for the reasons discussed previously. Given that the current expert guidelines strongly support the use of OST and psychosocial therapies, it is high time that a clinical trial of these approaches with physicians as patients, working with medical boards, is undertaken. Until that sort of evidence is available, it is probable that ABPT will remain the treatment of choice for most opiate-addicted physicians and that most will continue to do well in tightly monitored physician health programs.

Finally, it is important to examine the barriers to treatment that physicians face and explore why they typically are not referred for treatment until their addiction is quite advanced. There are many reasons for this, with probably the most commonly reported one being what Berge et al. (2009) have described as a "conspiracy of silence" within the medical profession. These authors quoted a study of more than 1,800 physicians, in which 17% of respondents reported knowing personally of an impaired or incompetent physician within their circle in the past 3 years, but only two-thirds of this group reported their incompetent colleague to a relevant authority. They also noted that physicians working in small practices were less likely to report an incompetent colleague, so that among doctors who were aware of an impaired or incompetent associate, only 44% of those in a solo or two-person practice filed a report, compared with 77% of those working at universities or medical schools. What this reticence to report, or even to discuss their concerns with their colleague, often means, sadly, is that doctors frequently struggle in silence with their depression and/or substance abuse, as was the case with Dr. Ward. This denial and conspiracy of silence is frequently supported by healthcare institutions, who often cover up for incompetent physicians, as described in the case in Chapter 6, and these physicians tend also to be supported by spouses and family members who do not want to report their impaired loved one in case this affects his or her job and the family economic stability. Importantly, one of the core skills that has recently been added to the national training curriculum for all residents is the ability to approach and discuss with a colleague concerns they might have about their colleague's mental state or capacity to practice. It is hoped that this will at least give physicians more tools in the future to be able to assist one another.

There are numerous other barriers, however. One that is specific to drug dependence is that if the workplace, as was the case for Dr. Ward, is the source of the substance, this encourages long hours of work and increasing professional isolation. Addicted physicians are very hard to recognize because they continue to function at high levels for a long time and their problems only tend to become obvious when their performance is markedly impaired. Table 5–1 includes a list of signs and symptoms that might be detected in the workplace for physicians who are addicted either to narcotics or to alcohol. It is clear from this list that those who choose alcohol, which is a substance that is not available in the workplace, are likely to be detected in the workplace earlier in their addiction because their signs and symptoms are more obvious.

Center et al. (2003), in an important consensus statement on physician health, examined a number of other professional and institutional barriers to physicians seeking help for themselves. They noted the following issues as important barriers:

1. Thirty-five percent of physicians do not have a regular source of primary healthcare, which means that they use fewer preventive medical services, and in particular, physicians' use of mental health services was low. Barriers to care reported in the literature included lack of time, lack of confidentiality, stigma, cost, and fear of documentation in a medical or insurance record.
2. Practicing physicians with psychiatric disorders have traditionally encountered overt discrimination in medical licensing, hospital privileges, health insurance, and malpractice insurance. Center et al. cited examples of medical boards focusing excessively on specific psychiatric diagnoses rather than on potentially impaired professional abilities. Although these discriminatory policies are gradually changing, there is still significant implicit bias held by many against physicians who have psychiatric disorders, and this can lead to administrative and licensing de-

TABLE 5–1. **Signs and symptoms of alcohol and opiate dependence that may appear in the workplace**

Signs suggesting opiate dependence	Signs suggesting alcohol dependence
Abnormal pupils	Alcohol on the breath
Sweating	Slurred speech
Agitation	Unsteadiness
Mood swings	Tremor
Frequent absences or bathroom breaks (to self-dose) or addition of long sleeves (to hide track marks)	Impaired memory and concentration
	Erratic performance
	Poor hygiene and dress
Poor record keeping regarding drugs	Lateness
Long hours of work and volunteering to deliver drugs	Unexplained absences
	Sweating
	Irritability
	Poor social behavior

cisions that are detrimental to the physicians. Not surprisingly, physicians with psychiatric disorders tend to do all they can to avoid contact with medical boards and similar institutions. It is also common, for instance, for physicians who are patients to pay cash out of pocket, rather than to make a claim on their insurance, just to ensure that their insurer does not know that they are seeing a psychiatrist.

A final concern held by many physicians relates to their career progression and professional advancement. Although there are few specific data on this issue, the medical community can be quite small, and rumors and stories move around easily. This is potentially important when physicians are changing jobs, and perhaps moving to somewhere they are not well known, where a referee's casual adverse comment can do considerable damage to their chances of gaining a new position.

References

American Psychiatric Association: Diagnostic and Statistical Manual of Mental Disorders, 5th Edition. Arlington, VA, American Psychiatric Association, 2013

American Society of Addiction Medicine: The ASAM national practice guideline for the use of medications in the treatment of addiction involving opioid use. June 1, 2015. Available at: https://www.asam.org/docs/default-source/practice-support/guidelines-and-consensus-docs/asam-national-practice-guideline-supplement.pdf?sfvrsn=24. Accessed January 26, 2018.

Berge KH, Seppala MD, Schipper AM: Chemical dependency and the physician. Mayo Clin Proc 84(7):625–631, 2009 19567716

Center C, Davis M, Detre T, et al: Confronting depression and suicide in physicians: a consensus statement. JAMA 289(23):3161–3166, 2003 12813122

Crowley R, Kirschner N, Dunn AS, et al; Health and Public Policy Committee of the American College of Physicians: Health and public policy to facilitate effective prevention and treatment of substance use disorders involving illicit and prescription drugs: an American College of Physicians position paper. Ann Intern Med 166(10):733–736, 2017 28346947

Hughes PH, Storr CL, Brandenburg NA, et al: Substance use by medical specialty. J Addict Dis 18(2):23–37, 1999 10334373

Johnson K: Physicians who use marijuana are "unsafe to practice." October 29, 2012. Available at: http://www.medscape.com/viewarticle/773544. Accessed January 28, 2018.

McLellan AT, Skipper GS, Campbell M, et al: Five-year outcomes in a cohort study of physicians treated for substance use disorders in the United States. BMJ 337:a2038, 2008 18984632

Merlo LJ, Campbell MD, Skipper GE, et al: Outcomes for physicians with opioid dependence treated without agonist pharmacotherapy in physician health programs. J Subst Abuse Treat 64:47–54, 2016 26971079

Rose JS, Campbell M, Skipper G: Prognosis for emergency physician with substance abuse recovery: 5-year outcome study. West J Emerg Med 15(1):20–25, 2014 24696748

Rose JS, Campbell MD, Yellowlees P, et al: Family medicine physicians with substance use disorder: a 5-year outcome study. J Addict Med 11(2):93–97, 2017 28067757

Skipper GE, Campbell MD, Dupont RL: Anesthesiologists with substance use disorders: a 5-year outcome study from 16 state physician health programs. Anesth Analg 109(3):891–896, 2009 19690263

Substance Abuse and Mental Health Services Administration: Behavioral health trends in the United States: results from the 2014 National Survey on Drug Use and Health. Publ No SMA 15-4927; NSDUH Series H-50. September 2015. Available at: https://www.samhsa.gov/data/sites/default/files/NSDUH-FRR1-2014/NSDUH-FRR1-2014.htm. Accessed January 28, 2018.

Yellowlees PM, Campbell MD, Rose JS, et al: Psychiatrists with substance use disorders: positive treatment outcomes from physician health programs. Psychiatr Serv 65(12):1492–1495, 2014 25270988

CHAPTER

6

Disruptive Behavior and Life as a Ponzi Scheme

"THANK YOU FOR allowing me to interview you, Mr. Stillman. I really appreciate this and understand that your son's story is likely to be painful for you to tell, so do take your time. I want to confirm that you are in agreement to my taping this conversation so that I may make sure that my final piece to be published about your son is accurate and that my readers understand what happened to him, and why."

Beth Masters, the young investigative journalist, looked up to confirm that her interviewee, a fit-looking man in his 60s with a weathered bronzed face and short military-style haircut, wearing a smart polo shirt and casual slacks and loafers, was fully in accord. Mr. Stillman nodded his agreement and sat back in the comfortable hotel lounge chair, waiting for the interview to begin. He had secretly been dreading this interview but was determined to put on a brave face and to be as honest as he could about

119

the awful scandal that had enveloped his wife and himself after their son's death.

She continued. "I have done a lot of reading about your son, Dr. Brent Stillman, and about his accomplished and tragic life and career. Much of what I read came from some rather dramatic reports after his suicide 10 years ago, so do excuse me if some of the questions I ask are wrong, or are based, in your opinion, on inaccurate facts or situations. I will do my best to be as sensitive as possible and hope that between us we can work out an accurate story of his life, and his death. I know that you have never spoken publicly about your son before and that you want to do this one interview to set the records straight on the tenth anniversary of his demise."

Beth took a deep breath. She knew she had to get the beginning of the interview right and not cause even more stress to Mr. Stillman. It had taken a long time to convince him to be interviewed about the story that had captured national attention a decade ago. She wanted him to break his silence and to let him tell what he thought had really happened to his son. She decided to start gently and positively, rather than jumping in too fast. She wanted to understand why his son killed himself in a way that was so cruel to his daughters.

"So perhaps we could start at the beginning. Your son, Brent, was, I understand, a very brilliant student and athlete and from an early age stood out from his friends."

"Yes, he was," Mr. Stillman responded. "I can remember when he was only five that he was already reading far above his age. He also loved sports. He was able to literally hit a baseball out of our garden at the same age and seemed to delight in always pushing himself to do more than his friends, and at times more than we wanted him to."

Beth sat back in her chair and relaxed a bit. At least this was a good start. Mr. Stillman took a deep breath and continued to talk more about his son's childhood—a relatively nonthreatening topic. "Can you give me some other specific incidents that you remember—that stood out?"

"Sure. He had so many interests it was hard to keep up with him. He would take up something new like tennis, and then once he could do it well, he would lose interest and move on to the next curiosity. For instance, he always had lots of pets—we had a large house and as you know he was an only child, so I think we certainly overindulged him—and he would always have a favorite pet at any one time and then tend to ignore the others. But the next week a different animal would be "special" to him. We never quite understood what was going on. He was always close to his animals, almost like brothers and sisters, but then for no apparent reason he would lose interest and ignore the recent favorite. And then, when he was about 10, he suddenly lost interest in all of his pets completely and ignored them totally. At that point we just looked after his remaining cat, dog, and rabbit until they finally died, but it was as if they had never existed for him. In retrospect, given all the problems he had with relationships and addictions later in his life, I can see this early pattern of him being over-involved with the latest and greatest pet, and then abandoning it for an alternative animal, as an early sign of his later behaviors. He did the same with his friends from an early age—he would focus entirely on one friend for months, then they would do something that upset him, and he would never speak to them again and move on to befriend other children. He was always able to make superficial friends quickly and easily and seemed to be almost seductive in his relationships, even from a very early age. He would have other kids doing exactly what he wanted, whatever the activity, until they didn't, at which stage he would get angry and frustrated and move on to the next group of friends, activity, or interest. He was very frustrating to live with, and we often had other parents complaining to us about his tendency to upset their children. By the time he was 12 he had gone through all the neighborhood kids and he had no friends at all. We actually got him into counseling on the advice of his teacher, but he only went twice before refusing to attend any further, saying that the counselor was stupid and that she just wanted him to draw pictures of us, his family, which he refused to do. I wish we had insisted he continue, but we didn't. As usual, he got his own way and we took the path of least resistance. We never made him face the consequences of his behaviors, and that has always haunted me, that maybe we were to blame. But I know that other kids didn't behave like him in the first place, and didn't need to have consequences, so I've finally come to the view that his problems were mainly within him, rather than the result of our overindulgence." A long pause while Mr. Stillman reflected. "Likely a bit of both, I guess."

Beth listened intently and tentatively tried to move the conversation forward. She didn't want Mr. Stillman to get stuck on Brent's childhood when there was so much else of interest. "You mentioned his later problems with addictions. Can you tell me more about those?"

"Certainly." Mr. Stillman sat forward and started to choose his words carefully, trying to make sure he was accurate in what he said. "As I'm sure you know from the newspaper reports at the time, Brent turned out to be a brilliant student and excelled throughout school and college. While we thought his erratic behaviors and attitudes towards other people, his lack of long-term friends, and his high self-interest were really signs of him being an eccentric genius, it became clear halfway through medical school that this was not the only possible explanation."

"What happened then? Why did you change your mind?"

"I remember the lead-up to his first DUI. He was on a medical rotation and working long hours with a group of other students in a high-pressure academic unit. He felt that the other students were not contributing as much as he was and that he was more intelligent than them. In a situation where he was meant to be working as one of a team, he ended up having a big argument with another medical student and was then taken aside and confronted about his selfish attitudes by one of the senior physicians on the unit. I still feel guilty about this, as I know that at home we never made him face the consequences of his behaviors. It was always easier for us to move on and ignore his lack of tolerance for others. This was really the first time in his life that he had ever received a dressing-down and direct negative feedback for his arrogant and insular attitude. I remember that he phoned me and said he planned on leaving medical school. That he thought all doctors were stupid. That they didn't understand that he knew best what to do. I had never heard him so angry and aggressive. So he left the hospital ward where he was meant to be working and went to a pub and just got drunk. It seems that he had done this a few times previously at medical school when things didn't go his way, but this time he drove home and was stopped by the police with a blood alcohol level well above the legal limit."

"What happened next?"

"Well, we came to the rescue as usual. We paid for a fancy lawyer, and he ended up with just some community service and a fine. We passed it off as an isolated time. We didn't even consider he actually might have a drinking problem. He decided to continue medical school, although he always harbored a grudge against internal medicine physicians for confronting him, and, to give him his due, he stopped drinking altogether and finally qualified with high honors. He still had no friends. I think this whole episode may have been one of the reasons he went into surgery. He found that the surgeons who taught him at medical school were much less interested in his attitude, and more focused on patient outcomes and the technical aspects of surgery, which he liked. He told me once that they seemed more tolerant of eccentric or difficult behavior in their colleagues, and some of them were almost proud of it."

"Do you mean you think he actually went into surgery partly because he thought he might fit in better there?" Beth suggested.

"Yes. I think that is probably true at one level," Mr. Stillman replied, "although I have no doubt that he mainly went into surgery because he thought it was the specialty where he could stand out the best and really prove how good he was. There is no doubt that he loved operating, and he found the adulation that he received from thankful patients very rewarding. Maybe that was another addiction of his—on the positive rewards of his specialty. So you probably want me to tell you more about his surgical career."

"Thank you, Mr. Stillman. I understand that it was in residency, and after that as a junior trauma surgeon, that his problems really started to show themselves."

"Sadly, that's true. I think he found the pressures of surgery, and the expectations of his mentors and the high workloads, too much, and he started drinking and sporadically taking Valium and other tranquilizers as a way of escaping when he wasn't on call or working. He didn't even try to hide this behavior. He talked about it like it was normal. I can remember him telling me that he felt he was invulnerable and that he would never have problems with these substances because he could always stop them when he had to work. In his practice, he worked shifts—often 24 hours at a time—but with time off in between, so this somehow all made sense to us at the time, or at any rate we wanted to believe him and convinced ourselves what he was saying was true. In support of what he said, he continued to do really well professionally and gained several rapid promotions. Anyway, this continued for several years, and we now know that he started using more and more of both drugs, and finally, almost inevitably, he had another DUI, this time when he fell asleep at a traffic light driving home late at night after an evening out. This was early in his relationship with Claire, whom he eventually married. A really sweet girl who I thought would be good for him and would help him reduce his use of drugs and settle him down."

"What happened with this second DUI?" Beth asked.

"It was interesting," Mr. Stillman continued. "Not what I expected after his first DUI led to few consequences. This time the medical board got heavily involved, so while the courts fined him heavily and banned him from driving for a year, the medical board made it clear that a second DUI by the time he was only 35 was a serious problem. They were especially concerned when it came out that he was due to be working a shift only 4 hours after the time of his DUI and would have been intoxicated at work had he not had to spend the night locked up in jail."

"I didn't realize that he was drinking at work. That never came out in the newspaper articles after his death. Do you know more details?" Beth asked.

"I'm afraid I do. I have no idea how often he had been drunk, or affected by tranquilizers, at work, but I'm confident it had to have been a number of times because I know both I and my wife had talked to him about it several times when we would find him the worse for wear at home. He always had some sort of excuse for his intoxication—usually a fight with a colleague, or something going wrong that he blamed on others. Nothing was ever his fault. I'm sorry that his colleagues at the time didn't report him, because they must have noticed his abnormal behavior on occasion, but I've since learned that some doctors are very unlikely to report each other. Anyway, that whole episode was a very sad and expensive time for us because he had huge legal costs to try and battle the courts and the medical board, and to keep the whole event as quiet as possible so that his surgical career wasn't ruined by too much publicity. We were legally successful at the time, although I look back now and wonder if this may have led in part at least to him ultimately killing himself, because he never really had the treatment or therapy that he clearly needed. As a result, he was able to keep on the self-destructive path he was already on and avoid any consequences for his behavior, but we didn't understand that at the time."

Mr. Stillman stopped talking, took a sip of water while he marshaled his thoughts, and then continued. "You may be wondering what happened, and how he managed to cover up his use of alcohol and drugs and not be adversely affected by his poor relationships with other physicians. He was a junior surgeon at the time, and his career was taking off. He used to come and see us and proudly tell us how pleased his senior colleagues were with his technical results, and how good his surgical statistics were—how many lives he had saved. I have no doubt he was a good surgeon, because how could his career have progressed so well despite him having so few friends or colleagues who liked him? He used to complain about other surgeons and on several occasions told us about arguments he had had with them. I think there were actually a couple of times that his colleagues went as far as reporting him for being overly aggressive and patronizing, but as far as I know those complaints never went anywhere. I know that he was always a very difficult person who never attempted to look at issues in any way except from his own perspective, and I just assumed that his colleagues would not have put up with him had he not been an excellent surgeon. Anyway, he would tell us how he was able to do the most difficult operations and how he loved the buzz of operating in emergency situations. One of the psychiatrists who wrote a report for the medical board at the time described him as having a version of the "hero syndrome," where people promote their capability and importance to the level where it seems that they have been performing heroic acts, even occasionally initially dramatizing or exaggerating situations so that their actions can seem even more substantive and heroic. Certainly that would fit some of the stories he told us, where patients came to the hospital after a major trauma and he believed he was the only one capable of saving them. He made sure that the patient's family knew that at the time so that they ended up glorifying him after surgery. He was always very proud of the positive reports he received from patients, but this behavior made him very unpopular with some of his colleagues. He didn't seem to care about that, however, although it did mean that relatively few were prepared to help him when he finally got caught out and his behaviors were reported in the media.

"I'm sorry. I'm digressing. His whole story is just so complicated and tragic." Mr. Stillman stopped and seemed to inwardly regroup, before continuing.

"After his DUI, and given his lack of popularity, many other hospitals would have fired him I suspect, but he was valued as an excellent surgeon, and the hospital stuck with him and kept him on. After all, maybe he brought in so much money the hospital was prepared to look the other way. I really don't know why they didn't do anything about him. He was lucky not to lose his medical license from what his lawyers told me, and they were able to argue that he should only receive a public reprimand as it had been a decade since his first DUI and he managed to get a number of supportive medical and psychiatric reports considered. The whole episode was very stressful for him and lasted for over a year. In the end, and despite paying a fortune for lawyers, he couldn't avoid the consequence of many people hearing about his public reprimand, and its being posted on the medical board Web site. For the first time in his life, he began to lose confidence. He was furious and very frustrated with the whole medical system, which he told me had punished him unfairly. He never acknowledged that he could have been a potential threat to his patients with his alcohol and drug use, and that he had actually been very lucky not to have lost his license. He remained convinced that he could control himself and that everyone else should just keep out of his business. He was especially humiliated by one of the psychiatric reports requested by the medical board that described him as having a "narcissistic personality disorder" and that noted that his behavior regarding his colleagues and coworkers was indicative of him being a "disruptive physician." He read all about these terms and was furious when he found descriptions that said that such individuals were often also thought to be "jerks" and were widely disliked within the workplace environment. So sad, and so difficult for me to think about even now. Obviously, I've read about this personality style and his disruptive behavior since, and the descriptions do match him all too well. Such a brilliant mind in such a twisted personality. Such a waste. In retrospect, the other tragedy here is that yet again he was not referred for treatment or therapy. His lawyers were focused entirely on trying to preserve his license and his reputation, and no one except us seemed interested in trying to get him some help. I tried hard to make this happen, and I confronted him on this. We had a huge fight and he ended up refusing to talk to me for about a year."

Mr. Stillman sat back, quietly reflecting on his son's life. Beth said, "But I understood from the media reports that he actually did very well following this DUI. That he kept sober for several years and that his surgical career really flourished during this time."

"That's true, and I give most of the credit to Claire—she was a wonderful wife. She is still a very loving and forgiving person, even now after all that she and the children have been through. I think Claire kept him together for several years, and of course having the two girls also helped—he adored his daughters from the moment they arrived and tried to spend as much time with them as he could. That's why I cannot understand how he arranged his death so that they would find his body. It was all so cruel and awful. Unforgivable. They were still young and impressionable, and he scarred them for life. Imagine being teenagers and finding your dad dead from carbon monoxide poisoning in his car in the garage after you came home from school…completely unexpected. And then reading a letter from him, addressed to them because he knew they would find him, that he had left literally pinned to the front of the suit he was wearing."

Mr. Stillman stopped talking abruptly and sighed deeply. Almost on the verge of crying. "Telling them that he loved them but could no longer look after them as life had been so difficult for him. That he had often been badly treated and poorly understood and that they would be better off without him. Just awful. Such an angry and tragic end. As usual not taking responsibility for his actions. Instead blaming others. And with such long-term consequences for so many people. Look at us here, for instance, still talking about it 10 years later."

Beth shifted in her chair. She knew much of the story so far from the newspaper reports at the time, and the melodramatic headlines about the brilliant 47-year-old surgeon, at the top of his career, who had suddenly killed himself. There was initially no obvious reason. It was a complete surprise to his surgical colleagues, or so they were quoted as saying in the papers. Then the follow-up stories of his long-standing prior hidden history of alcohol abuse and disruptive behavior, and finally the most extraordinary events when at the coroner's inquest, a second "wife" with two young children she said were his came forward and claimed he had been living with her for over 8 years.

Beth decided she would try to uncover more of the backstory to the scandal following Brent's death. "So how do you think all these early career and personal problems led to his death more than a decade later?"

Mr. Stillman looked at her quizzically. "I guess you mean how could an apparently successful surgeon with a loving wife and two daughters live a double life with a second family for so many years. You know, no one will ever really know. I read all the reports at the coroner's inquest, and then there was the massive legal battle over his estate because he had left two wills, with the most recent one relating to his 'hidden' wife and family. As I am sure you know, a year after his medical board public reprimand he changed jobs and moved to different cities to continue his career in a place where his background was not so well known. He seemed to devote himself to Claire and his daughters, but he never made any friends, and I know that whenever we visited him, he would always be complaining about the neighbors, work colleagues, and almost anyone else he came into contact with. Always blaming them for his perceived grievances. Never taking any responsibility for the arguments he had with everyone who did not agree with everything he did or thought. Claire was just amazing. She would follow him around and clean up after him when he had been rude or obnoxious to someone. Everyone thought she was both long-suffering and wonderful. We still do. He didn't deserve her."

Beth interjected, "What do you know about his second family, Ruth, and his other two children?"

"Obviously we've gotten to know them well over the past 10 years. It is interesting how similar Ruth and Claire are to each other. Both are very forgiving, warm, and caring and were devoted to him. They have both had to deal with finding out about each other. It has been hard for them, but over time they have gotten to know each other and now realize they were both deceived and both were victims. But I think you want to know how all this happened."

"That's correct. It is rather extraordinary," Beth added.

Mr. Stillman continued. "Most people's reaction to the story is that it can't be true. How could anyone live such a life of deception? How could two wives be so completely fooled for many years? Those people don't understand Brent. How he was so convincing and believable. How he was so good at fooling people. How he did this for so many years. It's sad to say it about my own son, but he simply could not be trusted on almost any issue. He just did what he thought would be best for him, and part of that was taking risks and evading the consequences of those risks. I think he almost enjoyed the whole process of risk taking and found it exciting. It was like he was eventually addicted to thrill-seeking behavior, such as was necessary to fool his two wives and families, and his colleagues. His dual life was somehow similar to the life he had when he was originally addicted to alcohol but kept this hidden at work."

"That's interesting. I hadn't thought of the story of his two separate lives as being somehow related to his addiction. But it makes sense. I can see how that might have given him a constant sense of adventure. How almost every day he had to make sure that his wives did not discover each other. How he had to keep them both separate from his work, which gave him the excuses of long hours and many conferences, to be away from each of them regularly each week," Beth responded.

"Correct. But as I've said, he was highly intelligent and really quite sociopathic, although I would never have admitted it while he was alive. He only cared about himself ultimately, but he was very cunning. Both Claire and Ruth are really quite similar, and, as I've since found out, he set up his two families in similar ways, which helped him evade being found out for years. Both of them are excellent mothers and homemakers—both focused primarily on their children. Neither was particularly interested in his career except for what he told them about it—how he was regularly saving lives and how patients loved and praised him. He never told them about the many interpersonal problems he had at his work, and how unpopular he was with his colleagues, except to complain about them. Neither Claire nor Ruth wanted to go to hospital events or attend any of his conferences—and both accepted his explanations that all these would be boring for them, and mainly technical in nature. In both families he ran the finances and did the bills, so that stopped his wives from looking into any documents that would have given him away. They both had a separate housekeeping account, but neither of them ever saw the phone records or bank statements, and they were both OK with this. He drove his own car, and they were not allowed to drive it or use it, and that is where he kept anything he had to hide from either of them. He told them his car was exclusively for him to use for work, and whenever he was with either of them he used their cars for anything related to the family so that he always had a place, the trunk of his car, where he could hide whatever he wanted from either of them." He paused. "They were both very trusting. Really giving and caring but dominated by him. They completely believed what he said to them."

"It just seems extraordinary that such a relatively high-profile person could have kept a double life going like that for so many years," Beth commented.

"True. And he fooled me completely. My wife and I thought he only had one wife and family—Claire, Virginia, and Lilly. I can see now how he managed it though. He took no interest in or involvement with any friends or people who lived in the neighborhood. In fact, I remember being with them one weekend when I bumped into a neighbor. We got talking, and when the neighbor found out who I was, he gave me a piece of his mind about how rude and arrogant Brent had been to him on several occasions over little things that meant nothing. He explained at length how no one in the locality wanted anything to do with him. He had a dreadful reputation as an intolerant, difficult, and domineering individual locally. They liked Claire and the girls but were frankly pleased when he was not around— which of course was often. I've since found out that he behaved the same way with neighbors at the home he shared with Ruth, and that he also did the same at work, which led, of course, to his eventual downfall."

"So what did happen? Why do you think he ultimately decided to kill himself?" This was the key question for Beth. She had already learned a lot more from Mr. Stillman than she had expected. She had enough material, combined with her interviews of Claire, Ruth, and some of Brent's surgical colleagues, for an excellent article. But no one had really been able to answer this question. No one had been able to get inside Brent's mind at the time of his suicide.

Mr. Stillman had thought a lot about this issue. He and his wife had felt guilty about Brent's death ever since, especially the awful way it had occurred and the effect on Brent's daughters. They had gradually come around to accepting what had happened over time, and as they found out more and more about their son's extraordinarily deceptive life, they felt easier and blamed themselves less. After all, he was the one who lived the life of lies, not them, even though they knew that they had enabled his behavior for much of his life. Mr. Stillman had finally decided that he was not responsible for Brent's behavior, and this had led him to look more objectively at what his son had really done, and possibly why. And he was finding that talking in this way to Beth, covering Brent's whole life, was actually quite a relief. Having his feelings locked up inside him for so long, and only being able to share them with his wife, had been difficult. In some respects, getting the truth out there would be good.

"I've thought a lot about why he killed himself." He continued, "And I've done a lot of reading as well as going to some meetings of Al-Anon, the support groups for families of alcoholics. I think the key issue with Brent, which we never truly recognized, was what the psychiatrist working for the medical board recognized. He had a narcissistic disruptive personality style, which was combined with a range of addictive and high-risk behaviors that changed throughout his life but that I'm sure were related. We all knew he had an addiction to alcohol beginning in his mid-to late twenties, but he always avoided treatment, and he never maintained sobriety, always relapsing after a year or so following a crisis. He always refused to continue with individual counseling and was very dismissive of any psychiatrists or counselors. It seems that he reverted back to drinking quite heavily in the last few years of his life, although very discreetly and carefully. As you know, at the time of his death he had a moderately high level of alcohol in his bloodstream, even though he had been at work all day. I'm pretty sure his continuing intoxication must have had an impact on him towards the end. He would have found it harder to juggle all the components of his double life, and he must have worried about being caught out again at work, which of course is what eventually happened and probably was the final straw that broke his back and led to his death."

Beth interjected, "I didn't know about that. What happened?"

"Well, because of his death, it was all hushed up, I understand, but one of his colleagues told me that his behavior at work had been becoming more and more unstable. In the year before his death he changed and was frequently late for work, was more disorganized, and started forgetting details of clinics and patients. You know, the simple routine things in a physician's life that are essential. He apparently also appeared increasingly distracted and irritable and was more aggressive and defensive with his colleagues than usual. He even came to work in a rather disheveled manner on occasion, as if he had slept in his suit the night before. A few of his colleagues knew of his background with alcohol problems years before, and several who worked closely with him had started to wonder if he was back drinking again, although they never smelled alcohol on his breath or thought he was overtly intoxicated at work. Anyway, to cut a long story short, I understand one of his surgical colleagues spoke to a psychiatrist colleague about him. He was advised to talk directly to Brent about his concerns and to ask Brent what was going on and if he needed any help. It seems that the surgeon tried to have this conversation with Brent, but Brent instantly became very angry, started shouting at him, and walked out of the coffee shop where they were talking. That happened on the day before his death, and from what I understand the surgeon was very affronted and upset by what had happened but did not have time to get back to anyone about the incident. After all, this was not the first time by any means that Brent had exploded in a conversation with a colleague."

Beth was listening intently. "My goodness. How difficult a situation for the other surgeon. You never think of how to confront people like your son in this sort of circumstance. Good for his colleague for trying, though it sounds like it may have inadvertently, at least partially, led to the final tragedy."

"I think that's right, although I'm sure if it hadn't happened then, something else would have happened fairly soon afterwards. There were so many other things going on, and I think Brent was in a slow downhill spiral. I had also noticed a change in him that last year. He seemed more depressed and irritable. He told fewer stories about adoring patients, and I even heard him being critical of them, which was something completely new, as their praise of him was what he usually boasted about. I actually took him aside and told him I was worried about him 6 months before his death but he brushed me off completely. But the biggest change was in his attitudes towards Claire, Virginia, and Beth. He just seemed to no longer even talk about them. He had always been domineering and somewhat critical of Claire, and that just became more obvious and occurred more overtly when we visited on a couple of occasions. He had previously treated his daughters really well, though, and had seemed to love and cherish them. Now he became angry and irritable with them. He constantly told them that they couldn't have things that they asked for, such as new clothes or payment for school trips. It was as if he were having financial problems, yet we thought that he should be fine of course, given how hard he seemed to work as judged by the hours he was absent. He became easily angry at them and blamed them for putting pressure on him. He started to tell them that they were spoiled and didn't deserve to be going to their private schools, and that if they didn't behave better he would take them out of school. On one occasion, so Claire told me, she thought he was going to hit Virginia just because she complained that she hardly ever saw him and he couldn't come to a school play she was in.

"Apparently that incident led to Claire starting to ask him more about his absences and putting pressure on him to spend more time with his family instead of being away so much, and that must have made life more difficult for him. Claire told me later that she had started to worry about why he was gone so much. She had never checked up on him before, but she was growing concerned. Things just weren't adding up. It was so sad seeing his relationship with his wife and daughters deteriorate. Of course, I now realize that he really did have financial problems and was getting into major debt by having to pay for four sets of private school fees and cover the increasing costs of children as they became older. And at the same time, he wasn't doing anything like the amount of surgery that he told both families, because he had to see them at the agreed-upon times he had carefully planned of course, so his salary was just not sufficient to pay for all his expenses. The banks had started to come after him and were refusing to lend him more money, despite his having refinanced both the family homes 2 years before his death. I found a number of letters from two banks in the trunk of his car, from which it was clear to me that neither bank knew about the other and that he had been juggling money, and debts, between them, and an increasing number of credit cards, for several years. I took those letters and went to see the banks after his death. He owed about half a million dollars in total and had no possible way of paying off such debts, so my wife and I decided that we would cover those to reduce the scandal and to enable his four children to stay in their homes, at least for a while. It's tragic when you think of it. Even after his death we were still covering for him."

Mr. Stillman sighed and sat back. Seemingly exhausted from the story.

Beth decided to summarize the conversation. "So it seems he had a very difficult personality and that there was a series of things happening all at once that led to his death. He was drinking heavily, was most likely depressed, had large financial problems, and was possibly going to be in trouble at work, and his carefully laid deception with both wives was in danger of being uncovered. But why would he be so angry at his daughters that he would die by suicide and leave a note blaming them for his death?"

"We're never going to know unfortunately. He never should have gone into medicine. His personality was just not suited to it. His lifelong cravings—to be praised and glamorized, to be seen as important, and to be able to deceive people and successfully take risks—and of course his use of alcohol and drugs, were a combination of weaknesses that were too much. And in going into surgery, he found an environment that at least initially tolerated him and his disruptive self-centered behavior. It was his lifelong habit to blame everyone else for his own problems. I think even at the end that was what he was doing. He was likely blaming his four children for being the cause of his financial problems, and he saw his financial difficulties as the reason why he had to drink. Really his whole life was like a massive Ponzi scheme. There were so many interrelated components that all collapsed when just one or two weakened. And in his case the core weak links that broke were his finances and his drinking for which he always refused to get proper long-term treatment. So being confronted by a colleague about possible drinking, for the third time in his career was just too much for him. He was ultimately a fragile person who couldn't take responsibility for his behaviors."

Commentary

Brent's tragic story raises several issues of importance, the most important of which is the concept of the disruptive physician, usually an individual with a severe personality disorder, and how best to manage or assist such doctors to reduce the very negative impact that they can have on their colleagues, and ultimately on the broader healthcare environments they work in, and on patient care.

This is probably the single most difficult issue in the whole area of physician health and the one that is least well dealt with by most health organizations. Every major health system has several such physicians, who in the past were usually tolerated but who now are being recognized increasingly as individuals with personality disorders whose behavior can no longer be tolerated. The question becomes, why were they tolerated in the past, and what can now be done with and for them, and can this situation be changed? And an equally important question is, how can the disruption and distress that they cause be prevented, and is it possible to recognize them earlier and either prevent such individuals from getting into medical school or, as that is never going to be entirely possible, at least recognize them earlier and intervene at that stage? Finally, how best can these individuals be assessed and treated, to make sure they do not continue to slip through the system for many years, as Brent did?

The other issue of importance is the tendency of disruptive physicians to have dual diagnoses. Such people frequently have addictive behaviors and substance addictions as well as a tendency to become depressed, and potentially suicidal, as they age. This is when they gradually become confronted with life, as happened with Brent, and with their own increasing inability to succeed at the rather grandiose level that they have always believed was possible.

What is disruptive behavior, and how does one define a disruptive physician? Brent was called a "jerk," which is often exactly how such individuals get labeled. They are difficult, unhelpful, selfish, and rude, with minimal thought for those they work with. Such behavior in physicians makes for interesting television shows and is significantly exaggerated in importance and frequency in the eyes of many who see the world through such a media prism. Doing a Google search of "difficult doctor" returns 4.3 million hits, while a search of "disruptive doctor" returns over 700,00 hits, and "disruptive physician" over 550,000 hits. There is no doubt that there is a massive amount of information about this topic and interest in it, yet at a practical level there continues to be great uncertainty about how to manage both the behaviors and the individuals who exhibit such behaviors. It is important to note that disruptive behaviors may be exhibited by anyone working in healthcare and are certainly not unique to physicians. Physicians, however, have a disproportionate impact on patient care, so when they are disruptive, the effect is greater.

Rather than try to make up a definition, it's pertinent to refer to several excellent, very detailed documents that have reviewed this whole issue in detail and which generally focus on the topic as a major component that has to be addressed to ensure a culture of safety. These include an excellent, very detailed guideline from CPPPH (2017), as well as the American Medical Association (AMA) Code of Medical Ethics (AMA 2018) and the AMA 2009 report on physicians with disruptive behavior (AMA 2008), as well as a Joint Commission report in 2008 (The Joint Commission 2008) on behaviors that undermine a culture of safety. Taken as a whole, these four documents cover much of the medical literature of relevance to this topic.

The CPPPH guideline (CPPPH 2017) summarizes why this topic is so important:

> It is fair to say that many authorities and many disciplines are wrestling with the topic of disruptive behavior of physicians. The effort is necessary because of its impact on patient safety, organizational culture, regulatory compliance and risk management. It is also necessary in order to help physicians remedy those behaviors that undermine a culture of safety. To side step the issues and avoid engagement with a practitioner whose behavior is raising questions does a disservice to our patients, our colleagues and our profession. It may also do disservice to the physician, because the behavior may be a signal that he or she is suffering from a condition responsive to treatment.

The CPPPH guideline goes on to define a disruptive physician's behavior as

> a pattern of personal conduct, or even a single instance, deemed by peers to be outside of professional standards and detrimental to a patient, patient's family member, the health care team or the efficient delivery of health care services. The behavior may be physical or verbal; the behaviors may be overt intimidating behaviors (verbal outbursts, physical threats) or passive (refusing to perform functions related to appropriate patient care and patient safety, refusing to return phone calls, using condescending voice intonation). The behavior may or may not have affected patient care and patient safety. The fact that the behavior in question did not result in actual disruption of patient care does not change the fact that it is considered disruptive….It is both the way the behavior is received or perceived by the recipient and the effect it has that can determine whether the behavior is considered "disruptive," requiring a response from the medical staff.

There are many examples of disruptive behavior given in the literature, both single egregious incidents and long-standing continuing behavior. The classic historical example of disruptive behavior is the surgeon who throws scalpels across an operating room as a way of intimidating his team of assistants, but thankfully that is very rare in today's world. Other, more common examples include almost any form of intimidation or bullying, physical or verbal abuse, noncommunication, refusal to return calls or complete mandated tasks such as charting, frequent absences or unreliable attendance, physical contact or intrusive behavior, sexual comments or actions, property damage, threatening behavior, combative behavior, and inappropriate communications and sarcasm or demeaning comments, including via social media. Brent displayed a number of these, and not surprisingly, most of the complaints about his behavior and actions came from staff and colleagues over the years, rather than from patients, who frequently adore and praise disruptive physicians, even if they are not getting the best standard of care.

Why, then, do some physicians exhibit these clearly abnormal and self-centered disruptive behaviors? In Brent's case, he clearly had a lifelong narcissistic personality disorder (American Psychiatric Association 2013), but this was combined with an alcohol use disorder, with the consequences described and discussed in Chapter 4, and eventually with depression—illnesses that led to his final demise by suicide. In this way he was typical of many individuals who exhibit disruptive and abusive behavior and who themselves have underlying medical and/or psychiatric diseases or personality disorders that may affect their behavior.

The presence of a personality disorder in an individual is usually evident by early adulthood and consists of rigid, unhealthy patterns of thinking, functioning, and behaving, leading to difficulty in relating to people and situations. Ten different types of personality disorders are commonly recognized (American Psychiatric Association 2013), and Brent's primary psychiatric problem was his lifelong narcissistic personality disorder. People with narcissistic personality disorder typically have an inflated sense of their own importance, a lack of empathy for others, and a deep and continuing need for admiration, behind which mask lies a fragile self-esteem that makes the individual very vulnerable to criticism. They tend to believe that they are special and appear arrogant with unreasonable expectations of favors, often taking advantage of others, while at the same time being boastful of their own success and attractiveness and dismissive of others. Brent clearly met all these criteria, and because of his ability to avoid the need for long-term therapy and the consequences of his behavior, this led to his many years of problems in relationships, work, and eventually his financial affairs.

It is common for individuals with personality disorders also to have other psychiatric disorders, or dual diagnoses. There has been relatively little research examining the main groupings of diagnoses that are likely to underlie, or contribute to, disruptive behavior, although one small uncontrolled retrospective study of 54 physicians referred for disruptive behavior to the Florida state physician monitoring program (Merlo et al. 2014) has examined this issue. The authors found that of these 54 physicians, 41 (75%) had one or more Axis I diagnoses, and 39 (72%) had one or more Axis II personality disorder diagnoses. The primary Axis I diagnoses were adjustment disorder (30%), impulse-control disorder (30%), mood disorder (24%), and anxiety disorder (11%), while the Axis II disorders were overwhelmingly in Clusters B (often described as dramatic or erratic) (48%) and C (often described as anxious or fearful) (50%). The authors noted a number of major limitations of this study, including that most subjects were male and that the retrospective nature of the study precluded meaningful conclusions as to the directionality of the link between disruptive behavior and diagnosis. This may have been the reason for the large number of reported adjustment disorders, which may have developed secondarily. It is also very odd that none of the physicians were reported as having a substance use disorder, but by the nature of the monitoring program referral, such individuals may have been excluded. Table 6–1 lists diagnoses of psychiatric disorders likely to be seen in physicians referred for disruptive behavior.

The consequences of disruptive behavior are many, and some have already been mentioned. In Brent's case they were mainly interpersonal and ended up affecting other staff and his work environment. Merlo et al. (2014) have categorized the consequences as involving the work environment, staff, and patients (Table 6–2).

While the protection of patients, employees, practitioners, and other persons at the hospital is the primary concern of any health organization, and this series of consequences makes it clear how disruptive behavior can be seen to threaten the orderly operation of the hospital, the individual practitioner exhibiting disruptive behavior is also of great importance. As CPPPH (2017) has noted,

> The health of the practitioner deserves attention because experience has shown that certain individuals who exhibit disruptive and abusive behavior may have underlying medical and psychological issues that affect their behavior, and, if those can be effectively addressed, other forms of action may become unnecessary. It can prove helpful in the long run to make an initial assessment of whether there is an association between a practitioner's health (physical health and/or mental and emotional health) and his/her behavior. There should always be a consideration, first, of whether there is a possibility for a therapeutic intervention that might result in the

---

TABLE 6–1. **Psychiatric disorders likely to be associated with disruptive behavior**

Primary psychiatric diagnoses

Depressive disorders

Bipolar and related disorders

Anxiety disorders

Substance-related and addictive disorders

Intermittent explosive disorder

Personality disorders

Paranoid personality disorder: a pattern of distrust and suspiciousness such that others' motives are interpreted as malevolent

Narcissistic personality disorder: a pattern of grandiosity, need for admiration, and lack of empathy

Passive-aggressive personality disorder: a pattern of negativistic attitudes and passive resistance to requirements for adequate performance in social and occupational situations

Neurocognitive disorders

Mild cognitive impairment, delirium, dementia, or any organic brain damage

---

physician's willingness to modify behavior and to cooperate with monitoring that will document the desired change in behavior.

What, then, should be done about disruptive behavior, and how could Brent's final outcome, with many years of pain and distress beforehand, have been prevented? The Joint Commission (2008) has affirmed that such issues can be effectively addressed, and if done so, other forms of administrative action may become unnecessary. As a result, it has mandated that all health organizations' medical staff committee processes must provide for the need to assess, treat, and manage physicians who exhibit disruptive behavior. This is a role primarily undertaken by the medical staff well-being committee, also as mandated by the Joint Commission and described in Chapter 9. Although a detailed review of how to manage such physicians is beyond the scope of this book, the best practical guideline currently available is the Canadian *Guidebook for Managing Disruptive Physician Behavior* (College of Physicians and Surgeons of Ontario 2008).

This guide defines three different levels of disruptive behavior and then describes a detailed behavior management workflow process for each level:

TABLE 6–2.　Consequences of disruptive physician behavior

Work environment	Patients
Tarnished public image	Increased mortality
Increased litigation expenses	Medical errors
Increased staff turnover	Medication errors
Decreased communication	Adverse events
Team breakdown	Decreased quality of care
Increased tension and hostility	Greater likelihood of legal action
Distrust of leaders	Feelings of fear and abandonment

Staff
Fear
Confusion
Uncertainty
Increased peer pressure
Grief
Apathy
Burnout
Early retirement/relocation
Hurt feelings
Low morale
Desire for vengeance

Source.　Adapted from Merlo et al. 2014.

Level 1: A single significant episode or a few mild problematic episodes—discuss and counsel, keep records, and possibly make referral to well-being committee.

Level 2: Multiple significant episodes—strongly consider a well-being committee comprehensive evaluation and agreement for treatment and compliance monitoring, which may be internal or external.

Level 3: Multiple significant episodes and failure to respond to interventions—strongly consider taking administrative action by medical staff executive.

What the guide suggests is that reports of disruptive behavior at any level warrant a response by the medical staff even before an untoward outcome has occurred or been identified. This is very important because it means that someone like Brent would have been identified early in his career as a potential disruptive physician because his disruptive behaviors would not have been ignored. There would have been a process to deal with him and to intervene early. Tragically, that did not happen, and he was able to avoid the consequences of his behaviors and also avoid treatment or behavioral interventions that would have helped him.

There are many barriers that exist within health systems that prevent individuals who demonstrate disruptive behavior, or the disruptive behavior itself, from being addressed. In other chapters there have been many discussions of the individual barriers that prevent physicians or their families from self-referring, but with disruptive physicians such barriers are typically even greater. At an individual level, as is evident from the high proportion of individuals with personality disorders, these physicians are simply less likely to have insight into their abnormal behavior. They will tend to project their fears, anger, and anxiety onto others, which naturally makes them less likely to self-refer, or even to understand that they are different, are causing distress to others, or are potentially impaired as practitioners. So while the individual barriers to referral are heightened, so too are the staff and institutional barriers, as has been addressed by Merlo et al. (2014). These authors have described the following barriers:

> *Staff.* Fear of retaliation, fear of jeopardizing a colleague's career, intimidation, covering up of behavior, concern that reports will be ignored, a belief that physicians are untouchable.

> *Institutional:* Lack of policies to address the issues, fear of litigation, lack of documentation of disruptive behavior, concern about angering "top producers," failure to recognize the problem, fear of jeopardizing a physician's career.

All of these barriers are important, and in any individual case there is usually a combination of individual, staff, and institutional barriers working against reporting abnormal disruptive behavior or individuals. All need to be recognized and potentially addressed for what can easily become a conspiracy of silence within a healthcare organization to be reduced.

Brent did have a number of evaluations after his second DUI, but only because of his involvement with the medical board, and all ended up being adversarial. His outcome could have been very different had he had an evaluation early on, as a junior attending perhaps (or even ideally as a medical student), and an intervention from the well-being committee of the medical staff of his hospital. This might have included a treatment referral and monitoring over time of his treatment adherence, as well as his agreement to function within the code of conduct of the hospital so as not to interfere with the culture of safety of the hospital. Had this worked, there would have been no need for disciplinary action. Such a nondisciplinary and rehabilitative avenue could have avoided the time-consuming and costly adversarial situations that eventually affected Brent, and ultimately might have prevented avoidable harm to his career and his family, and of course, ultimately, his suicide.

References

American Medical Association: Report on physicians with disruptive behavior. 2008. Available at: https://www.ama-assn.org/sites/default/files/media-browser/public/about-ama/councils/Council%20Reports/council-on-ethics-and-judicial-affairs/i09-ceja-physicians-disruptive-behavior.pdf. Accessed January 28, 2018.

American Medical Association: Code of medical ethics. 2018. Available at: https://www.ama-assn.org/delivering-care/ama-code-medical-ethics. Accessed January 28, 2018.

American Psychiatric Association: Diagnostic and Statistical Manual of Mental Disorders, 5th Edition. Arlington, VA, American Psychiatric Association, 2013

California Public Protection and Physician Health: Policies and procedures for medical staffs and medical groups: behaviors that undermine a culture of safety. 2017. Available at: https://www.cppph.org/wp-content/uploads/2017/02/Behaviors-that-Undermine-a-Culture-of-Safety-2017-1.pdf. Accessed January 28, 2018.

College of Physicians and Surgeons of Ontario: Guidebook for Managing Disruptive Physician Behaviour. 2008. Available at: http://www.cpso.on.ca/CPSO/media/uploadedfiles/policies/policies/Disruptive_Behaviour_Guidebook.pdf. Accessed January 28, 2018.

The Joint Commission: Sentinel Event Alert, Issue 40: Behaviors that undermine a culture of safety. July 9, 2008. Available at: https://www.jointcommission.org/sentinel_event_alert_issue_40_behaviors_that_undermine_a_culture_of_safety/. Accessed January 28, 2018.

Merlo LJ, Sutton JA, Conwell T, et al: Psychiatric conditions affecting physicians with disruptive behavior. Psychiatric Times, 2014. Available at: http://www.psychiatrictimes.com/mood-disorders/psychiatric-conditions-affecting-physicians-disruptive-behavior/. Accessed January 28, 2018.

CHAPTER

7

A Sudden Disastrous Day

DEAR RICHARD AND YVONNE,

I feel I have no choice but to end my life and am doing so in the hope that you will take this letter and employ it in the way that I suggest below. Please use what has happened to me as an example to help prevent the same tragedy happening to the patients of elderly physicians who have continued practicing past the time when it was safe for them to do so. I now know, as a result of the recent tragedy that led to the suspension of my medical privileges, and which effectively ended my career in disgrace last week, that I have mild cognitive impairment, which may be the beginning of dementia. Some may think me weak, but I cannot face the inevitable investigations that will occur into my errors, and so I prefer to die.

I was diagnosed with this disorder very quietly and privately by Dr. Michael Sanders, a local neurologist, about 2 years ago, but I refused to accept his diagnosis and was convinced that he was wrong. I went to see Dr. Sanders with the intention of obtaining some data to prove to the hospital authorities, including Dr. Bartless, that their concerns about my capacity to practice were wrong. I fully expected all the tests and investigations to be normal. My intention was then to produce these results and use them to ensure that I could continue practicing at the hospital. I deliberately paid cash to see Dr. Sanders so that no evidence of my possible illness, or even any concerns about me, could ever reach my insurance company or potentially my employer. I attach to this note a 2-year-old letter from Dr. Sanders confirming his opinion about this diagnosis and advising me to stop practicing. I hereby give you permission to access any other medical records of mine that he may have. Mistakenly, in retrospect because of my refusal to accept this diagnosis, I threatened to sue Dr. Sanders if he attempted to report me to my hospital or to the medical board. As you know, it is very difficult to diagnose early dementia, and Dr. Sanders made his diagnosis on the basis of extensive cognitive testing and the presence of what he called some neurological "soft signs" despite a normal MRI of my brain, and normal general physical examination and multiple laboratory tests. I genuinely did not agree with, or believe, Dr. Sanders but now accept that he was right and wish that I had stopped practicing when he told me to, or ideally, about 2 years earlier, when Dr. Bartless first tried to tell me.

Let me tell you my story, and why I feel I have no choice but to kill myself, bearing in mind that I may not be completely accurate as my memory is not what it should be. I do now believe I have early dementia. My primary care doctor, Dr. Burlington, whose notes you may also obtain, also diagnosed depression precipitated mainly by your mother's tragic illness and death, and I have been taking antidepressants that I think have been moderately helpful for the past 2 years. I have been thinking of suicide on and off throughout that time and wanted to talk to Dr. Burlington about it, but he seemed to be content to just reorder my pills rather than talk about how I was feeling, and I was always too embarrassed to bring up these thoughts. At times he seemed more interested in the latest breakthroughs in cardiology, and we would talk about these during our consultations, rather than about me. I have had no one to talk to about losing Ethel except for both of you, and while I know you have been as helpful as you can, I think I should have gone to see someone, but no one suggested this and I think I just assumed I would get through by pushing myself as usual.

Anyway, over the past few years I have continued my cardiology practice, treating mainly outpatients. Last year I reduced my work schedule to 4 days per week, and stopped doing the various cardiac interventions that I used to do. I have been enjoying my practice, and teaching medical students and residents, and this has really been the main bright spot in my life since Ethel passed. I have been very lonely and isolated at home especially as I have been so far from you and the grandchildren. No one's fault, but you are both busy as you should be in managing your lives and the children. I have been unable to enjoy life since your mother passed away. It's just been so lonely. The house too empty—too quiet.

I had to finally face the fact last week that I was no longer competent to practice medicine, and cannot face the knowledge that it took my mistakes, and the unnecessary deaths of two patients, for me to understand this. As we have talked about on the phone, I had this one dreadful day in the clinic where everything happened at once and I just couldn't cope. We were short-staffed that day and I was the only attending present, but that is no excuse. To have two patients suddenly get really sick at the same time was bad luck, or so many observers might say, but I know that a few years ago I would have managed them fine. The reality is that last week I was a major part of the problem and I couldn't manage the two patients together.

I became completely flustered managing Brian Hammond, the first sick patient. He was a nice man that I have known for years who had chronic atrial fibrillation. I rushed my assessment of him because I was worried about another patient I had just seen, a fit-looking 25-year-old man, David Ryan, a new patient, who I thought might have cardiomyopathy because of his angina-like symptoms with exercise. Anyway, while the nurses did a full EKG on Mr. Ryan, I started my examination of Mr. Hammond in the next room, and to my surprise on that day his heartbeat was way too fast and I realized he was potentially very sick. I decided to get an IV running and start treatment on him prior to sending him to the emergency room, which was our normal practice. Unfortunately, I became confused, although I did not realize it at the time, and gave him the wrong dose of medications to try and slow his heart, despite one of the nurses questioning me. I became irritated with her in this urgent moment and pushed her aside and drew up the medication myself. Immediately after I injected the meds I had drawn up, he collapsed and coded, so I then had to oversee the resuscitation attempt, which, as you know, failed. This all took quite a while, and I literally forgot about Mr. Ryan in my distress as the nurses, and then the ambulance officers, told me that I had given Mr. Hammond 10 times the required dose of his meds. I can remember calculating the dose but did it for the wrong medication. I was completely distraught. I had literally killed him through this error. I went into the staff room and remember being in tears and very distressed and angry with myself. I had never done anything like this in my life, and when the nurse brought me the EKG from David Ryan to look at, I was not thinking straight. I hardly even glanced at it, dismissing her so I could be alone. I told her the EKG was fine and he could go home. Looking back, I was in no state to make any decisions. I was very upset and felt suddenly completely clinically out of my depth. The clinic manager had already spoken to me about my error with Mr. Hammond and informed me that the coroner and hospital administration were being informed. She said she had called for one of the hospital cardiologists to come and take over from me and told me that I was to take the rest of the day off.

You know the follow-up story, as it was all over the newspapers last week. Mr. Ryan went home and took part in a basketball game that afternoon. Partway through the game he suddenly collapsed and died on the court. I had been right. He did have a cardiomyopathy, and it was obvious on the EKG I had ordered that same morning. The same EKG that I had hardly looked at, and the same patient I had not gone and reviewed in more detail after my initial examination. He should have been admitted to the hospital when I saw him, so his was the second death that I was responsible for on the same day. Not surprisingly the families of both men are suing, and both are demanding to know why a 79-year-old cardiologist was the only doctor on duty in the hospital outpatient clinic.

By the time you read this I will be dead. I genuinely thought I was safe and able to practice medicine, despite having been told otherwise, but I was wrong. I hope I did a reasonable job and made good decisions in the clinic when I could take my time and go carefully, which is what happened most of the time, although I cannot even be sure of this. Appropriately the hospital has arranged for all my patients to be reviewed by an independent cardiologist to check my practice broadly. Whatever is found from this review, it is clear to me, and to all my colleagues, that this tragedy shows that I could not any longer manage a difficult combination of circumstances, which is of course what we train all doctors to do. I now know that my memory impairment was the most likely reason for this and wish I had taken note of the test results from Dr. Sanders, or at least had not been so arrogant as to threaten to sue him if he released the results to the hospital.

I would like you to take this letter and give it to the hospital, the medical board, and the coroner and ask them to try to prevent this sort of tragedy occurring with other physicians. I now think there should be some sort of evaluation of all physicians as they get older, a bit like a repeat driving test, to make sure that if they wish to carry on practicing they are cognitively able to do so. I know many of my colleagues will disagree with this, but I am living proof that had this happened, three tragedies, the death of two patients, and my suicide, would likely have been avoided.

I am so sorry to have made you suffer through my obstinacy and my insistence on continuing to practice medicine when I was not fit to do so. I am going to join your mother and hope that she will understand and forgive me. I love you both.

Dad

Dr. Colin Bryant signed his suicide note, picked it up, and looked around his comfortable living room for the last time. He had been happy living here. He looked briefly at the row of photographs on the mantelpiece as he slowly walked toward the door, absentmindedly still carrying his pen as well as the note for his children that explained everything about why he was convinced that he, a 79-year-old cardiologist, deserved to die.

The large gold-framed photo in the center of the group of himself and his dear wife, Ethel, who had died 3 years before, took pride of place. It had been taken many years ago when they both were looking forward to a long and full life together. What a wonderful person, friend, and life partner she had been, and how he missed her. The loneliness of recent years had been excruciating, and the only way he had survived was by throwing himself into his work, until last week, when that had all gone wrong. In the photograph, taken over 50 years before on the proudest day of his life, when he had graduated as a physician from Harvard Medical School, he saw her sweet smile and her twinkling eyes. She was so full of life back then before she got sick. What an awful time she had had dealing with the ravages of ovarian cancer. Her pain was so difficult to manage. The hospice nurse visited often and tried so hard to relieve her suffering. Her pain and distress that went on for over a year, before she finally succumbed. His longing for Ethel and sadness with what she went through was overwhelming for him.

Then there were several photos of his two children, Richard and Yvonne, both of whom emailed and called regularly, having made their lives several states away. What gifts they had been to Ethel and himself and how he missed not seeing them more. Such wonderful caring adults now, both in their late forties with their own families, his six grandchildren, ages 8 to 19, who met with him on Skype when they had time. They all seemed so busy, but when they were able to connect they were all loving. Somehow he felt disconnected to them right now. He knew they would be so disappointed in him when they found out what he had done, and how his medical career had ended in tragedy, for the patients involved, and in humiliation for him. How awful. He just hoped his mistakes would not reflect on his children adversely. Richard, being an internal medicine physician, might understand somewhat better, and that is why he had mainly written the details of the suicide note with his son in mind, although he thought that Yvonne, who had always been more sensitive and caring than her brother, would be more forgiving.

On the walls beside the fireplace hung several of his awards and honors, achieved and received throughout his long and sterling career in cardiology. He could see his framed board certification, awarded after he had completed his residency in New York. What an experience that had been, to learn cardiology from the greatest physicians in the country, and then to have the honor of passing on his knowledge to countless medical students and residents over the course of his long career. He looked at the award beside the certificate. In some ways this was his greatest achievement, and the distinction of which he was most proud, "Teacher of the Year— Awarded for the tenth occasion to Colin Bryant, M.D." What a night that had been, just 5 years ago. No other faculty member had won so many teaching awards from the residents. Not even close. And to have won it at the age of 74, when most of his medical colleagues had retired several years previously. He couldn't in his heart of hearts believe that he had suffered from mild cognitive impairment at that time, but that is what had been alleged, and that he finally had realized was accurate.

He wondered why that diagnosis, often a sign of the early onset of dementia, struck such particular fear in physicians. Why was it that they couldn't tolerate the thought of any level of cognitive impairment, when this was so common? Was it simply that many doctors, like him, didn't want to ever retire and that the loss of their intellectual capacities was a threat to this aim? What an irony that a diagnosis like that could finish a medical career without a single abnormal laboratory or radiological abnormality being found.

He looked at himself in the mirror above the mantelpiece and thought he looked fit for a 79-year-old. The only physical evidence he could see of any change in his health was his gradual aging in the many family photos. He had always been proud of his physique. Just over 6 feet in height, and never more than 200 pounds, although in the past few years he knew he had shrunk and become slightly bent forward somewhat. He still had his usual proud head of well-groomed gray hair that overlapped his ears in the fashion of 40 years ago. He had always dressed smartly in conservatively styled suits and gleaming leather shoes. Ethel used to tease him by suggesting that he must have been born wearing a tie. He sighed at this memory, admitting to himself that he had always wanted to look like the perfectly presented physician, whether at work or in a social situation.

He shook his head and quietly moved on toward the large bay window. He walked slowly, dressed in his best suit, blue and white pinstripes as ordered by Ethel a decade ago, and his hospital "uniform" since. This suit had always been kept in immaculate condition with regular dry cleaning at weekends so that he could have it available when he was doing teaching rounds in the hospital 2 days per week. He much preferred the suit to the scrubs he wore the rest of the week when he was in clinic. He knew that the students all joked that he was old-fashioned, but he didn't mind, as he had always believed that you should look smart if you wanted to be smart. Dr. Bryant was a man who liked routines and regular habits, more so in the past few years, and he admitted quietly and only to himself that being dressed the same for work at all times was also somewhat easier and less confusing than having to choose, and then clean, new clothes each day. For Dr. Bryant the outfit that he had chosen to die in, a beautiful set of pinstripes set off by the brightly polished black shoes, a glistening white shirt, and a red silk tie, was how he felt a cardiologist should really look like.

As he stopped to look out of the windows to see the houses in the street opposite him, he grimaced. What a grouping of mediocre homes now took up the view he and Ethel had had for so many years. He looked at the gray concrete street and the group of houses, all different styles and from differing periods, that now impinged on his garden and his privacy. The especially ugly one on the left side of the group had come first, way back in the 1980s, designed by an architect who won awards at the time but whose love of steel and concrete pipes and flaps meant that the house had always reminded him of the contents of a junkyard. What a shame they had had to look at this for almost 35 years. He tried to think back to what had been there before this horror and could just vaguely remember open fields and an old farm that had long ago been demolished. He surveyed the scene sadly and realized he really couldn't remember which houses had come first, or exactly when, even though he had spent a lot of time fighting the council to try to stop the building. He knew that he used to know all about them, but just couldn't remember these sorts of details anymore.

Finally, he arrived at the front door and turned around to look back into his home of over 50 years. He paused to take in his last view of the interior. He knew it was rather tattered and worn and that whoever bought it after his death would most likely renovate it completely. But he loved it, and he knew exactly where everything was. It had been perfect for him and Ethel and had been just the right size to entertain numerous groups of new residents at the beginning of each year, for many years, as had been his tradition until Ethel became ill. The blue lounge chairs where he and Ethel had spent many evenings reading quietly together, across from the small bar in the corner where he kept his favorite bottle of Laphroaig malt Scotch whisky, always replaced and available for him to have a "short shot," as Ethel had playfully called his occasional drink. Next to that was the sideboard, a family heirloom that he had not opened since Ethel's death. That had been her prize possession and contained their precious silver service, used only at Christmas and on special occasions, and their valuable cut crystal glasses and Royal Doulton china dinner plates, all wedding presents that he could not bear to look at, never mind use. He recalled that all of the contents of the sideboard were willed to Yvonne and hoped that she would like them as much as her mother had.

He could see the kitchen through the doorway on the far side of the room and noticed the white boards his daughter had hung up with simple instructions for him to follow to make his breakfast. Below them he saw that all the cupboards and drawers had large labels on them so he could easily find what he wanted. How frustrating he had found it to not be able to cook as easily as he had been used to doing throughout his life. At least the microwave had been a blessing. It was so much easier to cook a whole meal at one go than to remember all the ingredients and cooking requirements for the sorts of meals he and Ethel used to cook. He knew his short-term memory had been gradually getting worse at home, but it was only recently that he had had to accept that this was not just a home issue, and that the same had been occurring at work.

Dr. Bryant turned around and thumped the door in defeat. He knew he could not practice medicine anymore after such a disastrous day that had ended his long and fulfilling career in disgrace. He knew that the hospital had been right to suspend him last week. He looked distraught at these thoughts, and clenched his fists in frustration, his face tight and distressed, almost tearful, wondering why this had all happened. Why had he been so stubborn and continued working when so many people had told him he should stop? What was it about him that had led him to continue to practice, when he now realized he was demonstrably unsafe? And how could he ever make up for the people he felt he had effectively killed last week? How had he gotten to the stage where he could see only one way out?

He walked out the front door, not looking back. Dr. Bryant was focused on his final walk, about 20 yards across the front path and into his large garage by the side door. He had been planning the next 10 minutes all week and had made up his mind to end his sense of hopelessness and pain soon after he was sent home from the hospital by Dr. Bartless, the kindly but also guilt-ridden chief medical officer. Dr. Bartless felt that he was partly to blame for the major medical mishaps that had occurred, and Dr. Bryant's subsequent suspension. He had told Dr. Bryant that he probably should have stopped him practicing at least a year or so before but had not done so. Dr. Bartless convinced himself that he could keep an eye on him and make sure he didn't have any complicated cases. He had tried to be kind by allowing him to continue practicing so that he did not suffer yet another loss on top of Ethel's death. He had initially planned to just let him practice for a few months after the funeral, but time got away and he had not been watching over Dr. Bryant like he had planned.

Dr. Bryant entered the garage and saw all his preparations in place. Like everything in his life, he had researched his method of suicide carefully. He recalled that doctors had a higher suicide rate than equivalent nonphysicians and that the main cause for this was that doctors were simply better at killing themselves than other people and used their medical knowledge to that effect. He fully intended to be successful in this final act. He had thought of overdosing or of self-injection but didn't want to take the risk of being found before he was dead. He didn't want to shoot himself because, first, he had never owned a gun and, second, it was very messy, and he didn't want to die with parts of himself spread widely around his garage. He decided on hanging after checking out multiple Internet resources and finding that this method was both quick and relatively painless, as well as likely to be successful. He had been surprised when he put "how to hang yourself" into the search engine that the first few links were all to places like the national suicide hotline and similar organizations. Clearly, he was not the first person who had done this type of research.

Dr. Bryant shook himself to clear his thoughts and looked around the garage. He saw the strong rope he had tied to the rafters that ended with his perfectly tied noose about 9 feet off the ground. He briefly remembered his love of sailing when he was a medical student and how he learned to tie numerous types of knots at the time, although this was another interest he had forsaken once he had qualified as a physician. To make sure he tied this knot correctly, he had also looked up Web sites instructing how to tie a hangman's noose. In the end he had found very easy-to-follow "how to" video instructions on the Web, which he had followed successfully. He was rather pleased with himself at succeeding in this simple learning task, especially when he reflected that he was using the same approach to learning that many of his students from the millennial generation used. Maybe he was not quite as impaired as he thought. Next to the noose was his garden stepladder, an old and faithful wooden 8-foot ladder, still in good condition, that he had used for years, mainly to clean out gutters. He knew that he had to climb about 6 feet above the ground for the drop to be sufficient and for his neck to break immediately. He had done all this research a few days previously, and once he had bought the rope from the local hardware store and set up his place of death 2 days previously, he had felt calmer. His decision was made. There was no going back. He had spent the last 2 days tidying his house, listening to old but familiar music, cleaning up his finances, and writing several drafts of his suicide note. Although he had exhausted himself, he could not sleep. He felt he was becoming emotionally numb. He just wanted to stop feeling so empty and sad. This was the end of the road for him, and all he could do now was see if his final act could help other colleagues avoid what had happened to him. He was confident he had done sufficient research and that his suicide would be successful.

Instead of going directly to the ladder, he sat down in his well-worn navy leather chair that had been in the shed since time immemorial and that he had used for many years to examine his beautiful butterfly collection. He had built up this collection beginning in his teens. Ethel had taken up this hobby with him over the years, which led to lots of weekends hiking together to gather new butterflies. They had spent many happy summers hunting with nets and then proudly displaying their specimens in glass cabinets placed all around the inside of the garage. This was not primarily a garage for cars, although he did put his car in sometimes; it was his place of peace and escape, where he could examine and study his magnificent collection of butterflies—a collection he had made in his role of amateur lepidopterist, and long-term active member of the local entomology society, and that was willed to the local museum, which would be receiving it sooner than they had expected. He had been fascinated by entomology ever since he studied it prior to going to medical school, and he had decided that he wanted to die with his butterfly collection as his last view on earth before the noose snapped his neck.

After looking briefly at his favorite butterflies, and setting them aside for the last time, he decided to move on to his last task before climbing the ladder. He was beginning to feel calm and even more determined, focused on becoming free from what had become a horrifying life a week before—a life that had been based on his service to patients and his commitment to the medical profession but that had culminated in tragedy and would end with his lonely and thoroughly planned death. He sat back in his leather armchair, relaxed, and picked up his carefully written and considered suicide note, to read it one final time to be sure he was completely comfortable with it, and that it said what he wanted. He hoped that there might be some good that would come out of his demise and that even in death he would help others.

Having read the note, Dr. Bryant carefully folded it and put it back in the envelope addressed to his son and daughter. He sighed and took a last sip of his scotch, setting the crystal glass down on the small table beside his note. He stood up slowly and stretched as he looked around the garage. He could see the camping gear, garden tools, and old paint cans from projects he and Ethel had done together over decades. He noticed the thick layers of dust everywhere, as he had not touched anything in the garage in the past few years. He climbed his wooden ladder and steadied himself by holding a rafter in his left hand, while he put the prepared noose around his neck with his right hand. He made sure the knot was at the back of his neck, well centered, so that it would break his cervical vertebrae and spinal cord without any difficulty, glanced briefly at the box of his prize butterflies hanging on the wall, and stepped off the ladder.

Commentary

Dr. Bryant's tragic story is, sadly, not unusual. A very sad finish to a lifetime of service and care that was preventable. He most likely had a combination of mild cognitive impairment (MCI) and depression, both of which led him to be unable to respond flexibly in an emergency situation, where rapid thinking and decision making are required, even though he may have appeared to be cognitively competent and capable of handling most routine day-to-day medical work. As a consequence, his actions in the scenario led to disaster and revealed his lack of continuing competence to function as a physician, in a way that was both personally humiliating and medically appalling.

Like the rest of the U.S. population, physicians are also aging, and a 2016 report from the Association of American Medical Colleges (AAMC) has shown that physician demand continues to outstrip supply, with over a third of active physicians predicted to be over 65 years within the next decade (AAMC 2016). The AAMC notes that as of 2016, physicians ages 65–75 already account for 11% of the active workforce, while those ages 55–64 make up another 26%.

The key question to consider is how society can best make use of the experience and commitment of the great majority of elderly physicians, many of whom wish to continue working past the normal retirement age. The great majority of physicians are likely to be physically and psychologically fit to practice into their 70s and 80s, and occasionally even longer if they wish. There needs to be a process to allow them to be able to do so as long as they maintain their fitness for practice, while at the same time ensuring that those physicians who become unfit to practice are able to cease working and retire with their dignity, reputation, and safety record intact. In an ideal world, Dr. Bryant would have been able to take a customized "fitness for practice" assessment that might have included checking his capacity to manage several difficult patients at once. This would have been a much more effective approach than the cognitive and neurological assessment he did receive. Had he been a surgeon, such an assessment might have included checks on his surgical manual dexterity, as well as his decision-making capability. Fortunately, such customized assessments are being introduced in some states and, for those physicians who pass them, can be extremely reassuring. Hawkins et al. (2016) have highlighted strategies to ensure competent care by senior physicians and the importance of this issue. They describe how any screening process needs to achieve a balance between protecting patients from harm due to substandard practice and ensuring fairness to physicians and avoiding unnecessary reductions in workforce.

There are numerous advantages gained from supporting those senior physicians who wish to continue working. These include their contribution to lessening the predicted physician shortfall that will occur over the next several decades as our population ages, and the continued availability of their medical wisdom and experience as teachers and mentors for more junior colleagues. At an economic level, society pays for much of their expensive medical education, so delaying retirement gives a greater return on this social and economic investment. Many senior physicians work in part-time voluntary roles as a way of giving back to society, or contribute to specific causes that could not otherwise have afforded their services when they were requiring payment. Finally, there is the matter of personal choice and preference, and many physicians who understand the old adage of "use it or lose it" make deliberate decisions to continue some form of practice at least part-time in order to maintain their own social, psychological, and cognitive health by keeping themselves socially involved and intellectually stimulated.

Dr. Bryant was determined to continue working, against the advice of colleagues, and had been to see a neurologist and had taken a battery of neuropsychological tests, which revealed that he had MCI. Unfortunately, he went into denial about the significance of this diagnosis and refused to accept it, or the consequences for him, as is not unusual. The neurologist, despite Dr. Bryant's threats to sue him, should have reported his concerns about Dr. Bryant's lack of practice capacity to the medical board, but he seems to have been ignorant of this duty, or to have been intimidated by Dr. Bryant.

MCI is a memory disorder with many possible causes, as outlined in a recent Mayo Clinic (2017) paper, that may or may not lead to dementia but that would generally make working as a physician unsafe. MCI is typically associated with loss of higher-level cognitive functions, such as forgetfulness of strings of facts, as occurs in conversations, books, or movies; an inability to make decisions and plan multiple steps to achieve a goal; and increased impulsiveness and poor judgment. Roberts and Knopman (2013), in a review of the classification and epidemiology of MCI, concluded that up to 5% of the general population have what is typically described as mild cognitive impairment. Given that this is a population baseline disorder, it can be assumed that up to 5% of physicians at age 70 also have MCI, and while some in that group will have undoubtedly retired or stopped practicing for one reason or another, many have not. This is an area that has not been widely studied, although a recent paper (Moutier et al. 2013) proposing more study of age-based screening cited Canadian data from Quebec and Ontario, suggesting that up to 22% of physicians over the age of 75 had gross deficiencies in their practice. Moutier et al. (2013) identified the risk factors that can affect physician performance as solo practice, lack of American Board of Medical Specialties board certification, practicing outside the scope of their training, high clinical volume, and health issues.

In terms of physician suicide, Dr. Bryant is not atypical, as most doctors who kill themselves are older than 50, and many are much older. Elder physicians, in particular, are likely to not have their deaths recorded as suicide either because colleagues deliberately fill in death certificates incorrectly or because they choose methods such as single-occupant motor vehicle "accidents" that are much less obvious than Dr. Bryant's well-planned action. Consequently, while death certification suggests 300–400 physician deaths by suicide per year, the number is likely higher, especially in the group of elderly physicians.

Like Dr. Bryant, these elder physicians, both male and female, frequently suffer many losses. In Dr. Bryant's case his primary losses were the death of his wife, his social isolation, the absence of his children and grandchildren, and, most importantly, his loss of memory and professional capacity. Ultimately, he became extremely lonely, with few continuing social supports, and was likely quite severely depressed, a condition that affects up to 5% of the elderly who live at home (Centers for Disease Control and Prevention 2017). Importantly, depression is also commonly associated with a degree of potentially reversible cognitive impairment called *pseudodementia*. In this situation, without treatment, an individual's thinking is literally slowed down, and the person becomes increasingly forgetful and less able to manage changes or make sudden decisions based on new information, as happened in the scenario.

Dr. Bryant's depression was only partially recognized and treated, and his primary care physician seemed to take an interest in his collegial activities rather than treating him like any other patient and focusing on his worrying symptoms of depression. His MCI seems to have been completely unrecognized by his primary care physician, partly at least because of Dr. Bryant's refusal to acknowledge this disorder. As such, Dr. Bryant's only active treatment was antidepressants, possibly at an inadequate dosage or without significant review of their effectiveness or otherwise, and he was not receiving therapy or any substantive inquiries about his state of mind, and especially about his possible suicidal intent or about his cognitive capacity. All medical students are taught not to be embarrassed or awkward about the issue of suicide and to always ask patients directly about suicidal intent. This is because we know that asking about this does not give patients the idea of suicide and that most suicidal patients are relieved to talk about these feelings, which they correctly recognize as abnormal. Had Dr. Burlington enquired about suicidality, Dr. Bryant might not have ended up dying by suicide, and his two patients might not have died.

As has been emphasized throughout this book, physicians are people and suffer the same baseline illnesses as the rest of the population, yet they have extra pressures and social obligations, positive and negative, and commonly work longer hours, and for more years, than nonphysicians. In particular, physicians become very adept at delayed gratification, working hard to achieve a short-term gain, while putting off the rewards from this activity to some future time. This also happens to many physicians as they face and enter the typical retirement years. As noted previously, it is common for some physicians to continue working into their 70s or sometimes longer, as they delay retirement and continue to work, often for professional, social, and personal fulfillment, either in a normal work role, frequently part-time, or voluntarily. For the great majority of physicians this gradual cessation of professional activities is completely fine. These individuals continue to contribute to society and continue earning, perfectly well, while slowly reducing their workload and frequently heading into retirement in their mid-70s, but it is not a good approach for the 5% or so of physicians in this age range who have conditions that cause some form of MCI. Statistically it is inevitable that larger numbers of these elderly practicing physicians will become gradually cognitively impaired while they practice, and that will lead to increasing numbers of tragedies for both patients and the physicians.

As was seen with Dr. Bryant, getting older can also be very isolating as friends and family pass on and physical and social capacities reduce, so the onset of depression in the elderly is also fairly common. Depression has associated memory and concentration difficulties, which for physicians who may already have some MCI, are additive and may lead to them being inflexible and unable to handle several crises at once, as happened with Dr. Bryant. The story described in this scenario, of an excellent physician who gradually and seemingly appropriately reduces his practice over a number of years but then suddenly has an unpredicted disastrous day where he cannot cognitively make a series of sudden essential decisions, is tragically not uncommon.

So what can be done about this? Dr. Bryant took the extreme step of asking for his situation to be publicized and reviewed by the appropriate regulatory authorities such as medical boards and those involved in credentialing physicians. In his suicide note he recommended a regular test for all physicians, rather like a driving test to maintain a driver's license. Many would agree with him, and there have been a number of attempts to implement such a process, generally through the mandating of certain physical or cognitive examinations at identified ages, typically commencing between ages 70 and 74 years, as well as several excellent policy reviews examining the issue in detail. A small number of health systems in the United States have actually implemented such policies, although this practice is certainly not widespread, and it's especially hard to define at what age any such policy should be implemented.

There seem to be four possible approaches to this problem.

1. Take no action and watch what happens as the physician cohort ages and increasing numbers of tragedies, such as affected Dr. Bryant, occur.

2. Screen all physicians when they reach specified ages, and on a regular agreed-on basis thereafter.
3. Mandate retirement at a specified age as part of a contractual enterprise agreement or as a legislated statewide arrangement.
4. Screen all physicians who may have some practice impairment and appear to be at risk whatever their age, as well as all physicians of a specified age, examining their competency and/or their fitness to practice in a customized manner.

California Public Protection and Physician Health (CPPPH) has published an excellent guideline on policies and procedures for age-based screening (CPPPH 2015), in which they have deliberately not taken a specific stance as to which approach is best, preferring to lay out the various options, one of which is the mandated screening suggested by Dr. Bryant. CPPPH reviewed much of the evidence for the interaction of increasing age, as just one of many risk factors, and a number of increasing parallel physician practice impairments caused by physical or cognitive limitations. They concluded that all hospital groups should implement some sort of age-related screening policy, as per the second approach above, that "applies equally to all members of the medical staff who have reached the specified age." As they noted,

> The rising number of physicians practicing later in life raises concerns about the potential impact of aging physicians have on patient safety. This is particularly troubling given the various studies finding when people reach their 60s and 70s, there is a significant and progressive decline in cognitive and physical skills. This is true of physicians as well. (CPPPH 2015)

There is no consensus on what age to screen physicians, but CPPPH has noted that mandated policies based on age, as per option 3 above, have been adopted by other professional groups, such as those representing airline pilots and law enforcement, who have mandatory retirement ages. A key argument in favor of age-based screening is that those with cognitive decline may either fail to recognize, or be unwilling to act on, their own decline, as happened in this scenario. This was demonstrated in a study by Davis et al. (2006), who reviewed the accuracy of physician self-assessment compared with observed measures of competence, finding that physicians had only limited ability to self-assess. So while it is clear that the competence of aging physicians is a major problem, and that a screening process for physicians like Dr. Bryant is essential, the issue currently is how to implement and defend a fair and standardized policy and practice against legal challenge, as has already happened in a number of instances. CPPPH

(2017) described an extensive, time-consuming, and expensive screening process for each physician who reaches whatever is the determined age. This process may have several components:

1. A full history and physical examination, including screening for alcohol/addiction issues, and tests of hearing and vision
2. Peer assessments of all core clinical competency areas—namely, professionalism, interpersonal and communication skills, medical knowledge, practice-based learning and improvement, patient care, and systems-based practice
3. Observations by others, such as nonphysician supervisors and risk management staff, conducted in a clinical setting
4. Assessment of cognitive function using recognized validated screening tests, undertaken by appropriately qualified evaluators

At the time of writing, a routine age-based screening process is still highly controversial (Melville 2017) and exists in very few health systems nationally. In those systems that do screen, most screenings include examinations of physical and mental capacity, the latter not always defined, and sometimes the use of structured cognitive assessments or hearing and vision tests, but few are standardized. Many groups have been put off by the highly publicized process that occurred at the Stanford Hospital and Clinics, where their experience of implementing, in 2012, a policy requiring all physicians age 75 or older to undergo peer evaluation of clinical performance and cognitive and physical testing every 2 years, was ultimately rejected by senior faculty members in 2015.

The next approach, which may appear to be superficially successful for some health systems, such as Kaiser Permanente, is to simply insist on a specified retirement age for all physicians. This means that while Kaiser does not have to deal with the problem of elderly physicians working for them, which resolves their internal concern and potential liability, their ex-physicians can of course continue working elsewhere, paid or voluntary, after they leave Kaiser, so the potential problem is not resolved but just moved sideways away from their jurisdiction. Other large physician groups around the country have similar contractual arrangements, and while these approaches will likely escalate in coming years as medicine becomes increasingly corporatized and small medical practices are reduced in number, there is no plan for mass mandated retirement ages, such as for pilots, to be applied to physicians.

This leaves the final option of screening individuals who demonstrate possible impairment, as well as all those physicians who reach a specified age, in a customized but standardized manner. Assessment of both groups of these individuals should ideally be managed and coordinated by physician well-being committees, as described in Chapter 9, and this is how Dr. Bryant should have been managed in his workplace.

The development of such customized, individualized, and standardized competency and fitness-for-duty assessments performed by experts who are less likely to be biased should be performed at a national or regional center. Some organizations and programs around the country, such as the University of California, San Diego (2018), Physician Assessment and Clinical Education (PACE) Program, have been developing these types of customized assessments as a better option than routine screening, as the competencies required to be a physician are highly variable. A surgeon needs a different skill, cognitive, and knowledge set than a pediatrician needs, while a pathologist has different needs than a dermatologist. In addition, there is no single battery of tests that can universally identify specific impairments in the many differing competencies that can be applied to all physicians to try to identify some form of generic impairment.

The issue of what to measure, and of how to assess physicians accurately and fairly, is difficult. Two approaches are typically used, *competency assessments*, which have been performed for many years, and *fitness-for-duty assessments*, which are a much more recent development.

The competency assessment is traditionally based on the six core competency areas defined by the Accreditation Council for Graduate Medical Education (ACGME)—namely, patient care, medical knowledge, practice-based learning and improvement, interpersonal and communication skills, professionalism, and systems-based practice. Competency assessments usually involve a series of standardized tests and are somewhat like taking a theoretical major board examination. They are mainly focused on proving that the individual is fit to meet the requirements of the academic competencies, but they do not tend to extend much beyond this, and they do not have a strong focus on the individual's health status. Competency assessments are useful for physicians who have had practice problems relating to their behavior or skills, or who have had professionalism lapses that have led to their licenses being taken away or restricted, but who want to be able to prove that they are now fit to practice once again, or when a medical board requires such evidence.

Fitness-for-duty assessments, as described by the UC San Diego PACE Program, are very different and can be useful for assessing senior physicians or any physician with significant health problems. Common elements of the PACE fitness-for-duty evaluation, as described by Bazzo (2017), are shown in Table 7–1. Had Dr. Bryant undertaken one of these assessments,

TABLE 7–1.   Common elements of the fitness-for-duty evaluation

Comprehensive medical examination

Toxicology screens

Neuropsychological testing

Neurological examination

Ophthalmological examination

Specialty medical examinations, including psychiatric

Functional assessment

Simulated procedural/skills evaluation in the physician's specialty

Chart reviews

Oral examinations

360-degree workplace survey

Source.   Bazzo 2017.

he would most likely have been asked to retire, a lifesaving decision for him and at least two patients.

It is clear that comprehensive fitness-for-duty evaluations make the most sense as an assessment tool for individuals such as Dr. Bryant. He would almost certainly have been asked to retire from clinical practice, but had he wished, he might well have been allowed to continue to teach and mentor junior colleagues and students, without any direct patient contact. Not surprisingly, these assessments are expensive, costing in many cases $8,000–$10,000 each, or sometimes much more if a lot of complicated procedural skills evaluations are needed, and currently most well-being committees and medical boards insist on the individual being assessed paying for the testing. Whether this will continue, or is fair, in systems where age-based testing is mandated is an interesting and thorny question and is likely to be litigated, but it seems that with the aging physician population the widespread introduction of such fitness-for-duty assessments is inevitable within the next few years.

References

Association of American Medical Colleges: The complexities of physician supply and demand: projections from 2014 to 2025. April 5, 2016. Available at: https://www.aamc.org/download/458082/data/2016_complexities_of_supply_and_demand_projections.pdf. Accessed January 28, 2018.

Bazzo D: Fitness for duty. Presentation at the 29th Annual Western States Regional Conference on Physician Well-Being, University of California, Riverside, May 24, 2017

California Public Protection and Physician Health: Assessing late career practitioners: policies and procedures for age-based screening. 2015. Available at: https://www.cppph.org/cppph-guidelines/. Accessed January 28, 2018.

California Public Protection and Physician Health: Guidelines for evaluations of health care professionals. 2017. Available at: https://www.cppph.org/cppph-guidelines/. Accessed January 28, 2018.

Centers for Disease Control and Prevention: Healthy aging. 2017. Available at: https://www.cdc.gov/aging/mentalhealth/depression.htm. Accessed January 28, 2018.

Davis DA, Mazmanian PE, Fordis M, et al: Accuracy of physician self-assessment compared with observed measures of competence: a systematic review. JAMA 296(9):1094–1102, 2006 16954489

Hawkins RE, Welcher CM, Stagg Elliott V, et al: Ensuring competent care by senior physicians. J Contin Educ Health Prof 36(3):226–231, 2016 27584000

Mayo Clinic: Mild cognitive impairment (MCI). 2017. Available at: http://www.mayoclinic.org/diseases-conditions/mild-cognitive-impairment/symptoms-causes/syc-20354578. Accessed January 28, 2018.

Melville NA: Age-based testing of physician competence stirs controversy. Medscape, 2017. Available at: http://www.medscape.com/viewarticle/878168. Accessed January 28, 2018.

Moutier CY, Bazzo DEJ, Norcross WA: Approaching the issue of the aging physician population. Journal of Medical Regulation 99(1):10–18, 2013

Roberts R, Knopman DS: Classification and epidemiology of MCI. Clin Geriatr Med 29(4):10.1016, 201324094295

University of California, San Diego: Physician Assessment and Clinical Education Program. 2018. Available at: http://www.paceprogram.ucsd.edu. Accessed January 28, 2018.

The Physician's Physician

DR. JOHAR STRUGGLED in her restraints, tied to the bed in the open cubicle, and screamed angrily at the passing nurse: "Come here immediately. I am not staying here. I am a physician. There is nothing wrong with me. I work at the United Hospital across town. I am a pathologist. Don't you understand? You cannot keep me here. I have my rights. My rights are right. What else is right? Why are you looking at me like that? Don't you know when to pay respect, you stupid foolish woman? I am a world-famous doctor and shaman, and savior. Savior, doctor, savior, doctor. Now come here and undo these restraints. There is no need for any of these. I have a thousand other doctors I am calling right now who will come and get me out of here. See, you can hear them coming. Here they come. They need me to save the world from cancer. Don't you see? You cannot keep me locked up in here. I have important works to do. I need to get to the hospital and finish my research tonight so that my cure for cancer can be published. It is nearly done. You are going to be responsible for thousands of deaths if you don't let me go."

The emergency department nurse looked sympathetically toward Dr. Johar. She knew her from the past when she had been admitted with a similar episode of acute mania, 3 months previously. She had since then, according to the hospital records, been diagnosed with a bipolar disorder, or what used to be called "manic-depression."

The nurse felt sorry for this eminent 45-year-old married physician, originally from India, who was now lying on a gurney, pulling her sheet off, ripping at her restraints, and screaming utter nonsense. She was obviously delusional and hallucinating and with no insight into her illness. She wondered how Dr. Johar, whom she had googled, had ended up in this state, especially given all the barriers she must have overcome to be appointed as an associate professor of pathology at the regional academic medical center. Dr. Johar's online profile presented a highly successful physician trained in another country who had worked hard to reach her current senior position. Her academic bio said she was a nationally renowned cancer immunology expert who held a number of federal research grants. Dr. Johar had two teenage children and was married to the CEO of a large IT company. The nurse felt embarrassed for Dr. Johar.

The nurse decided she needed to give Dr. Johar the medication ordered for her to calm her down and start her back on the road to reality. She dispensed 10 mg of haloperidol syrup into a small medication cup and approached Dr. Johar.

"Get away from me. I am not taking any of your poisons. How do I know what is in there?"

The nurse carefully offered the container to Dr. Johar. "Doctor, this will help you feel better. It's the same medication you had last time you were here. It is haloperidol, and it will calm you down. Here you are. Please take this medication."

Dr. Johar took the cup of syrup and promptly threw it on the ground, as the nurse rapidly backed away from her to avoid being hit. "See, that is what I think of your calming medications," she exclaimed angrily. Then her mood abruptly altered, and she suddenly shifted to an imploring tone: "See, nurse. I am fine. I don't need that. There is nothing wrong with me. Just let me go home. My husband is coming soon, and he will set me free, free, free. I just want to be free." By the end of this interaction she had changed again and was now singing and laughing at the top of her voice.

A month later Dr. Annie Johar sat opposite her psychiatrist, Dr. Sally Turner, as they reviewed what had happened to her over the past few weeks. Dr. Johar, no longer in scrubs, was wearing a beautiful sari, with gold trimmings over a dark-red-and-blue-flowered background. She had her shiny black hair tied back and was carefully made up with a painted dot in the center of her forehead, indicating her Hindu religion. She was wearing round tortoiseshell glasses that made her look professional. She sat forward in her chair looking intently at Dr. Turner, determined not to miss any of the conversation. They discussed what she could remember of being certified and forcibly admitted to the local psychiatric hospital for the second time in several months. She was embarrassed by her behavior, especially her almost undressing in public when she was feeling euphoric. Not surprisingly this had led to her being taken immediately to the emergency department. Her mania had gradually subsided over a 2-week period with a treatment regimen of lithium, a mood stabilizer, and risperidone, an antipsychotic, both of which she was still taking, although the risperidone dose had already been reduced.

Dr. Johar took a deep breath and continued talking. "I cannot believe what has been happening to me these past few months. I feel so unsure of myself at times. So vulnerable. I am beginning to accept that I have a bipolar disorder—I really have no choice because I was certainly psychotic this last time when I was manic. I was hearing guardian angels and choirs singing to me, telling me I could cure everyone of cancer. And I believed it. It makes me cringe to think of how foolishly I was behaving. The things I did and the people I offended. My children saw me when I was out of control and they are still treating me differently, even now."

"In what ways?" asked Dr. Turner, who was herself a refined-looking woman, with long blond hair neatly tied back. Dr. Turner was smartly dressed in her dark green suit and classic black pumps. She seemed confident and completely at home in her private psychiatric clinic with its ultramodern furniture and abstract art, the latter backlit and perfectly positioned around the large consulting room.

"Well, it's like my children have to constantly check on me. You know they have both repeatedly asked me if I am taking my medication. I have explained to them that I will take exactly what you say, unlike last time, when I thought I knew best and stopped my lithium soon after leaving hospital. They have been asking me what is wrong, and they look at me oddly. And my husband seems afraid to come near me. It is almost as if he thinks I am fragile. He is hardly touching me. It's as if he feels any stress or pressure may set me off again. I just wish he would start to treat me normally."

"I'm so sorry about that," said Dr. Turner, "but I think you'll find that they will all go back to their normal behavior once you've been well for a few months and they feel more confident about you keeping well. Unfortunately, they have been traumatized by your illness, just like you have, and it will take all of you a while to recover psychologically. Learning to understand and accept your illness is one of the issues we will focus on in our sessions over the next few months."

Dr. Johar responded, "You know, I still really cannot accept that I have an illness. It would be so much easier in many ways if I had breast cancer. Or a broken leg. I know I shouldn't do so, but I still actually blame myself for this. I must have done something bad in this life, or in a previous life, to be punished in this way. I know that as a physician with years of training I am sounding peculiar, and I shouldn't feel like this, but having a psychiatric illness like bipolar disorder is still somehow humiliating and makes me feel like such a failure. I cannot talk to my colleagues about it, although I know they all know what has happened to me. After all, it couldn't have been more public. I see them looking at me and wondering if I am sane or not, whether they can trust me or not. And this is still before I have returned to work. So far I have just had two short visits to my department to discuss my situation with my chairperson, Dr. Anderson, whom I know you have also spoken to. She has been very kind to me and has helped me get disability payments while I am off work. But even she looks at me slightly oddly as if she is trying to size me up and predict if I am going to suddenly do something bizarre."

"Well, the best thing you can do is work closely with me and ensure that you keep as well as possible," Dr. Turner said. "There will be a whole series of issues we'll need to discuss in the future in addition to how to make sure that your mood is as stable as possible and you are fit to work. In the meantime, the good news is that you have not had any difficulties at work and have not done anything that might have endangered patients, so there is no need for you to be reported to the medical board as long as you keep well. You know your colleagues respect you very much, and you have a great deal of support within your department, and Dr. Anderson did you a big favor by personally spending so much time double checking the pathology reports you had signed off on in the couple of days you had at work when your manic episode was just starting. She has reassured the hospital hierarchy that your judgment at work was unimpaired while you were there, and before your manic illness really took hold. You do not need to worry about your medical license, or any credentialing or other legal issues, as long as you keep yourself well and adhere to your treatment regimen. If your practice had been impaired and you had adversely affected any patients, we would have had no choice but to report you to the medical board. Fortunately, you have a good physician well-being committee at your hospital, and I'm collaborating with them. There will be a formal contract you will need to sign with them that will commit you to continuing to see me, and to follow up on any treatment you require to ensure you keep as well as possible, and we'll work through that process to make sure you are fully ready to go back to work."

Dr. Johar interrupted anxiously: "When will all that happen? I have looked at the physician well-being Web site and downloaded the sample treatment monitoring contracts, and they look reasonable to me. They certainly seem focused on my needs, although it worries me what might happen if I get sick again."

"We'll go over all of that together over the next few weeks," Dr. Turner responded. "I had a discussion with the chair of the well-being committee a few days ago, and she is very concerned about you and looking forward to meeting with you, hopefully in the next week or so. She is an internal medicine physician who has a great deal of expertise in addictions, and she has several psychiatrists and psychologists on the committee to help her, as necessary. She said that she planned on meeting with you with one of the psychiatrists on her committee so that they can get a good idea of what will be most helpful for you. In the meantime, please don't worry about them. Their job is to help you and to make sure that you remain well so that patient safety is assured and the hospital is appropriately protected knowing that all of its doctors are fully fit to practice."

Dr. Turner paused and then, seeing that Dr. Johar appeared reassured, continued: "So your job is to be a patient when you see me, and to work collaboratively with me as do my other physician and nonphysician patients. It is vital that you don't take any treatment shortcuts or attempt to treat or prescribe for yourself. Obviously, if at any time I think you are not fit to practice, you'll be taken off work, and if we have to limit your scope of practice, then the hospital would have to report that to the medical board."

Dr. Johar smiled back at Dr. Turner and replied in a somewhat uncertain manner. "I understand all that, but there are two issues that really worry me that I would like to focus on in particular over the next few sessions. They are concerns that I have that I just don't have answers for right now."

"Well, tell me what your concerns are, and we can certainly go over them," Dr. Turner replied.

"Thank you. I feel a bit embarrassed about them both, but they do worry me. And they are both related to me being a physician with a psychiatric illness. I feel I should know better, but I don't."

"It's OK, I promise you I have heard most things"

Dr. Johar looked down at her lap and spoke quietly. "Well, the first of them is about the bipolar disorder. There is so much stigma about having this illness, even among physicians. I have read about it a lot in the past few months, and I agree that I fit the diagnosis you have made, but I am still fairly ignorant. I only did 6 weeks of psychiatry as a medical student, and that was 20 years ago, so while I have read a lot about bipolar disorder in recent months, I really do not think I understand it very well. It is so different from pathology, which I have studied all my adult life, and I want to make sure that I get properly treated by you. I have heard so much about doctors getting poor treatment because they are assumed to know more than they actually do by their treating doctors. I want to make it clear to you that I would rather you treat me as you would any other patient and not assume that I have any useful knowledge about my illness. Is that possible? My main concern is the possibility of suicide. I couldn't bear to make another attempt on my life like I did 4 months ago. I was just so lucky that my husband came home unexpectedly and found me still unconscious but alive and was able to call an ambulance. So I want to try and understand what it is that might cause someone like me, a successful physician, to try to kill myself. Can we examine that, please? And in particular I really want to have a plan in place in case I get severely depressed again, so that I don't attempt to kill myself when I am in that state."

Dr. Johar paused and looked around the room, then took a deep breath and plunged ahead as if she had to take a risk in the conversation. "The second worry is my career. I think you will understand this issue because as a female physician you will have had some of the same problems. As a female academic, and as someone from another country, I have had to climb a lot of high ladders, and I want to progress further in my career, but I think this illness, this stigmatized psychiatric disorder, will slow my career. This is not just because I have had to take time off to be treated, but because of what people will think about me if, and when, they find out. I am really concerned about my license to practice in the long run, and about what my illness will mean when I have to reapply for credentialing privileges to work in my hospital. Or if I decide to change jobs and move to another hospital. What will happen then? Do I have to say what has happened to me? Will I be rejected? Do you have any experience working with people in my position? I fully understand that all of the systems that we have are mainly there to protect patients and to ensure that doctors are fully competent when they practice. And I agree with that approach. But what happens when a doctor has an illness that is hard to control and which may impair their ability to practice safely as a physician at times if their treatment is not fully working?"

"Those are both very valid concerns, and I really appreciate you bringing them up so directly," Dr. Turner replied. She continued: "I completely agree with you that they are important and that we must address them so that you can move on successfully with your life. Why don't we start with the first issue you brought up right now? Please tell me how you feel that being a female physician trained overseas has led to difficulties for you professionally. After all, one of the things we have to work on is how to manage any stresses that impact you so that you feel less vulnerable and can avoid developing another major mood shift in either depressed or manic directions."

Dr. Johar looked around the room, as if contemplating where to start and how to continue this conversation. Then she responded, "Let me tell you my story. I was born and brought up in Lucknow, in northern India, quite close to New Delhi. You have likely seen pictures of the Taj Mahal in Agra, which is just a night's train ride away and which I have visited several times. This is a very traditional part of India, with a lot of extremely poor people. I was last back in Lucknow 5 years ago, and it now has over 5 million inhabitants. Literally thousands of people sleep on the streets. There is so much overpopulation and poverty. It couldn't be more different from the United States. When I was a child, there were just a few hundred thousand people there. But Lucknow has a very well run and prestigious government hospital. As you know, there are many really high-quality health services and hospitals throughout India, mostly based on the British system dating back to when we were a colony before we gained independence. As the eldest daughter of a relatively well-off family who greatly valued education, I did well in school and then medical school, and was always able to work, and learn, at the Lucknow hospital during holidays and breaks from my education. In India medicine is a high-prestige profession, just like here, and like most of my classmates I automatically took all the American medical school step exams as I went through medical school so that I could always come here later in my career if I wanted. I was a very compliant young woman. I worked hard and received a lot of praise for my academic successes, which also made my family very proud. I had a most sheltered life in terms of boyfriends and lived at home whenever I was not doing jobs that forced me to live in the hospital, but this gave me more time to read and study, which I enjoyed. I was really typical of most of my female colleagues. We were expected to be self-sacrificing and hardworking and to help our family ahead of ourselves."

"So how did you come to move away and work in America?" said Dr. Turner.

"It's a long story, but to cut it short, when I was in my residency I had an arranged marriage to the son of a family who were friendly with my parents. I was quite a catch. A professional woman who came from a good family, who was training to be a pathologist, and who was well trained in all the home duties expected of a wife. My husband is a good man. My parents chose well, and they did give me the chance to turn him down if I really wanted to, but I knew they would be very disappointed if I did. Our marriage has worked out well. He is a computer scientist and completed his Ph.D. in machine learning and data analytics in Bangalore well before those topics became popular. He had always wanted to come to the United States, and soon after our marriage he took a job in California, where I was able to get licensed and work." Dr. Johar stopped and thought, looking out the window at the park nearby, before continuing.

"It was very hard at first. I was extremely innocent and was suddenly away in a foreign country, separated from my family, and starting a new residency again because my 2 years of residency in India had to be repeated here to let me get boarded. I got pregnant almost immediately, and, in retrospect, I can see now that the first year I was here, and after the birth of my daughter, was when I was first depressed. I didn't recognize it though, and neither did my OB/GYN. He was a nice man who just kept telling me to keep up with my work and that my tiredness and tearfulness were understandable given what I had been through. My husband was the same. He didn't know me very well but had been told I was able to do anything I set my mind to and that I always succeeded. So he just assumed I would get through OK, which eventually I did of course. It was so hard though, and I remember being terrified of holding my daughter, and even feeling quite dangerous towards her at times. You know, I managed to convince my husband to get help at home so that I could go back to work quickly, as I felt so unable to manage her. I can even remember wanting her to go away and thinking that maybe I could literally throw her out with the garbage at one stage." Dr. Johar burst into tears at this and sobbed, leaning forward, her head on her knees, in despair.

"I had such dreadful thoughts about my daughter at the time. I have never really felt close to her. I still wonder sometimes if I would have been better off without her. Don't get me wrong, I wouldn't harm her now, but I have had those feelings in the past. Just wondering how good it would be if we could both go to sleep together and never wake up again. I suppose I am sounding like I might have been suicidal postpartum, and I think that is true. Why didn't someone recognize how I was? You know, that whole year after her birth was almost wasted for me. I was back at work, but I couldn't concentrate, I was crying, I wasn't performing, and for the first time in my life I failed some exams—you know, the fairly easy ones you get at the end of each residency rotation. I was just not myself, and it must have been obvious to my friends and to my supervisors. My husband got frustrated with me and used to tell me to get myself together. I don't think either of us wanted to even think that I might be depressed, because that is such a stigmatized condition in India and was not something we even discussed or contemplated as a possibility. Why did no-one say anything to me? Looking back at family photos, I looked like a skinny ghost—always sad, not involved, looking away, just not the typical mother. You know, I don't think my moods have been really stable since. I just wish I could have been treated earlier; it would have made my life so much easier."

"What happened next? I imagine your depression resolved spontaneously eventually," Dr. Turner interjected.

"Yes and no. It is true that my depression got less, but I became very moody and irritable. Much more than I used to be. I think I probably had my first mild hypomanic illness when my daughter was about one. I can remember buying way too many clothes for her and throwing her a huge first birthday party, which horrified my husband. I literally invited all the neighborhood. I put invitations under everyone's doors and worked myself into a frenzy cooking and preparing far too much food. I felt wonderful and signed up for a new research project at work, which meant that I had to work late most nights, but that was OK because I didn't need too much sleep. I wrote two scientific papers to the delight of my attendings, who just encouraged me to do more. They had no idea I was unwell, and neither did I. I was just much more productive than usual. Anyway, as I told you last time, I have had a number of depressive episodes since, and probably one more high, which is why I have finally become convinced that I am bipolar. I have also spoken to my parents about this, and they told me about two aunts and a cousin who most likely have the same illness and who have all ended up in hospital in India a number of times. It is amazing how families can hide these things. I had no idea of any of this and had always been told that they were eccentric and liked going away on spontaneously unplanned holidays. Now I assume I have some degree of genetic vulnerability within me, and I wonder how that is going to affect me going forward, especially career-wise."

"You mentioned the difficulties being a female academic. What was your experience there?" Dr. Turner asked.

"That's important. I think it links into my bipolar disorder. Prior to coming to America, I always worked harder than anyone else, and always succeeded. Here, once I finished residency and was appointed as an assistant professor, I found it all much harder. Obviously I had my two children by then and my moods were unstable. But I was expected to do at least as much as all the other academics at work, and sometimes, in reality, more, because the academic expectations of women seemed higher. And this was in combination with my child-rearing role, where I wanted to see my children and spend time with them. I joined a "Women in Medicine" group and started regularly attending that. We used to discuss how to handle our lives—the big term everyone used was "work-life balance." To me it was just an acknowledgment that we had to do 150% of what our male colleagues did. I found it very hard to attend early-morning or evening meetings, for instance, and as that was when all the research and departmental meetings occurred, it was much harder to keep up. My husband was helpful and supportive of me, and of my career, but he also had a challenging job, and he just did not see it as his role to do his full share of the basic childcare and school things that as mothers we all have to do."

"What did you do? How did you resolve all these issues? Because I know you have done well in your career," said Dr. Turner.

"I think the most important thing I did was to get a good mentor who coached me how to set limits. This was one of my colleagues from the Women in Medicine group, Dr. Dinart, a pediatrician, who had her own family and who gave me lots of good advice. She suggested that all the young female pathologists discuss the situation with our chair, who has obviously also been through similar experiences. Over time we have set up a number of helpful changes in the department, with more flexible work time, covering for each other, and participating in writing groups, all of which have made our academic progression easier. It is just simply harder being a female academic because more is expected of you from many quarters. But I also try and understand my male colleagues, especially now that so many have wives who are also professionals with demanding work schedules of their own. They not surprisingly get upset if we try and ask for a lighter call schedule than them, or try to rearrange meetings during the day, when it may be less convenient for them, rather than after hours. They have lots of pressures too. I think a lot of this is just the expectations of modern medicine, and a group of competitive colleagues all trying to do their best in an increasingly complicated and litigious environment. I have spent a lot of time talking about the whole practice of modern medicine, and the pressures on physicians in general, with Dr. Dinart, and I still meet with her occasionally. In fact a year ago, she encouraged me to mentor a junior colleague in her department, which so far has been really rewarding."

Dr. Johar sat back and thought long and hard. Dr. Turner said nothing, just listening, as she knew from her own experiences how important these issues were for female physicians.

Dr. Johar resumed talking. "You know, it is really interesting how all these issues and stresses interact. It's so frustrating. Firstly, I am an Indian female working in a job that, despite 55% of doctors being female, I feel still discriminates against females because of the traditional requirements of a professional role. Then, I have my family—my daughters and my husband, and of course my family in India—and all the differing cultural expectations, never mind the need for me to be a mom and wife within the family. And then, I am unlucky, and I have a very stigmatized mental illness which most likely has a genetic cause and that is going to need very careful treatment and continuous monitoring, especially when I am depressed, so that I don't attempt suicide again. I cannot bear the thought of being psychotic again. I am so ashamed about all the awful things I did when I was sick. It is so humiliating. And finally, I am a physician, and somehow I'm expected to keep working really hard and know more about my illness than other people, yet the physicians I work with don't seem to be either able or prepared to notice me if I change. I wish they would talk to me and warn me if they see my mood changing. Maybe we can work something out about that as part of the monitoring agreement we talked about? And on top of all this, I am ambitious and I love my career. I enjoy studying and teaching and would like one day to be a full professor with my own lab and research team. I know I have the intelligence to achieve that as long as I can work out how to overcome all these other barriers first."

Dr. Johar continued talking, slowly and thoughtfully, putting emphasis into her words in an almost defiant way. "I know I am in a difficult position. I have been thinking a lot about this, and I've also been doing some reading. What it comes down to, ultimately, is learning to really accept that I do have this disease but that with treatment I can be all right. I want to talk to you about how to be more resilient in my life in general. I realize now that I had a very protected early life at home with my parents. I thought it was difficult, but it really wasn't. I just had to be prepared to work hard and keep focused. What I now need to succeed as a doctor is not just brains and hard work, or good medical skills, or good colleagues and a loving family, or even good luck. What I really need is to plan and be organized so that I keep well. I need to be resilient. To learn to be a survivor and to look after myself well so that I can look after my patients, and, of course, all those other people in my life. I wish resilience was taught at medical school. Perhaps they are starting to at some schools, because it seems to me that this is the most important solution for me. If I can learn how to be resilient and prevent the adverse impact of life's stressors on me, then I will be able to keep myself well, so I hope that is something we can work on together."

Commentary

Annie Johar's story is not unusual. About 2% of the U.S. population have bipolar disorders (National Institute of Mental Health 2017), therefore so do 2% of physicians. These illnesses generally have their onset in early adulthood, with at least 50% of patients who develop bipolar disorders having a strong genetic history in their families, so there is no reason to expect the prevalence of these disorders to be any less in physicians. The problem that Annie had, and one that many physicians face, is how to get appropriate good-quality treatment and keep oneself well while also continuing to practice effectively and safely, especially in our current era of increasing regulation and audit. In Chapters 3 and 5, I've discussed the difficulty that many physicians have in obtaining high-quality care for themselves, the barriers that occur as they try to seek help, and the fact that many physicians resist treating other physicians. In this scenario Annie meets with a psychiatrist who seems very used to treating colleagues, who does not assume they know more about their illness than an intelligent lay person, and who is knowledgeable and direct about dealing with her concerns. Dr. Turner was in no way intimidated by Dr. Johar and seemed very used to treating VIPs, or "special" patients, which is a skill in itself. What, then, are the skills and background that are necessary for a doctor who treats doctors, or a range of other potentially intimidating or socially high-ranking patients, and why are these not taught as a specific area of expertise? Every city has a few doctors who have developed a specific interest in treating VIP patients such as physicians. They usually come from backgrounds in primary care, internal medicine, addiction medicine (not infrequently with addiction in their own history), or psychiatry, but there is no curriculum in physician health, and most literally learn on the job as more and more physicians get referred to them over time. It is very strange that there is no specialized training to be a physician's physician given that anecdotal evidence suggests that most physicians either perform the role poorly or avoid it as much as possible. Not surprisingly, a physician who is unable to diagnose his or her own medical or psychiatric symptoms may well feel incompetent, and admitting this failure to another colleague may be potentially embarrassing. If this admission is then met with uncertainty, avoidance, or disbelief by a reluctant or unsure treating physician, it can only reinforce the physician patient's feelings of worthlessness and hopelessness and make his or her engagement in care as a patient much less likely.

The literature on the treatment of VIPs in medicine is fairly sparse because, not surprisingly given the patient group, there are no clinical trials or evidence beyond a series of anecdotal papers describing case reports and management concepts. VIPs themselves are usually described as being physicians, lawyers, politicians, businesspeople, celebrities, and the very rich. Alfandre et al. (2016) have reviewed the literature on such individuals and made a series of practical suggestions for their management, noting that the care such VIPs receive is different from the care received by other patients because VIPs tend to receive greater access to, and attention from, health care staff. The authors conclude that this care is not always of better quality if the staff are intimidated by the VIP patients. Alfandre et al. also note the traditional definitions of VIP in the health care world as "Very Important Person" and "Very Important Patient" but discuss how more accurate terms might be either "Very Intimidating Patient" or "Very Influential Patient," the latter two terms specifying that a VIP's personal characteristics might significantly change the clinician's approach, with deviations from the usual standard of care. Alfandre and colleagues resolved to use the term "Very Influential Patient" as their preferred nomenclature, focusing on influence as the key determinant of VIPs. In our scenario, Dr. Johar doesn't try to use her professional background to influence Dr. Turner and specifically asks to be treated as if she were any other patient who knows relatively little about his or her illness. So while Dr. Turner does not seem intimidated by her, it would be easy for Dr. Turner to excessively identify with her as a female physician who may have had similar career struggles, with a potentially adverse effect on her clinical objectivity. Alfandre et al. (2016) note that any physician treating another physician needs to be aware of such potential ethical concerns from overidentification and should be prepared to discuss them openly with the VIP.

The most common difficulty in the doctor-VIP relationship is the tendency to allow the VIP to determine his or her own treatment plan, which is often due to a combination of both intimidation and identification. While it's good to be "patient-centered," it's not good if a VIP's treatment plan denies the need for a primary care physician, as is the case with over 30% of doctors; does not include physical examinations or laboratory tests or drug screens; or leads the treating doctor to avoid using the routine diagnoses he or she might make in standard practice for fear of upsetting the patient. The most obvious example of the last mentioned is treating the physician who has a personality disorder, such as is described in Chapter 6, where it may be hard for the treating physician to be completely honest with the VIP, thus tending to support him or her in inappropriate treatments or lack of appropriate treatment.

Apart from intimidation and over-identification, there are a number of other potential traps for physicians treating other physicians who have psychiatric or substance-related problems. The first of these is privacy, and the potential difficulties or embarrassment that might occur if a physician is seen by someone he or she knows, perhaps one of his or her own patients, in a psychiatrist's waiting room. It is not uncommon for VIPs to be seen either early or late in the day before or after usual clinic hours to reduce this concern, or for them to be referred to other physicians or hospitals away from their place of work. Privacy is also important in terms of health insurance and payment issues. Many VIPs prefer to ensure that their insurance companies have no record of psychiatric treatment and consequently pay cash for consultations. Some VIPs may expect to be prioritized when there are only a certain number of appointments available and given extra access to their physicians via email or phone. All of these approaches may be reasonable as long as limits are set and the care of other patients is not impeded or adversely affected.

Dr. Johar's case also highlights the issue of how to treat physicians who have severe psychiatric disorders that may lead to psychosis (where she lost touch with reality and developed hallucinations or delusions), such as major depression, bipolar disorder, and even potentially paranoid psychoses. Such physicians need close monitoring and careful treatment to ensure that they remain safe to practice and, of course, keep healthy. However, for physicians with such disorders, the stigma and loss of a sense of their healthy self are often greater than what the general public perceives them to be, and the shame inherent in having a psychiatric illness, or in being unable to self-diagnose or self-treat correctly, is intense and can be life-threatening. Dr. Johar clearly showed this in her concern about her colleague's reactions to her and her uncertainty about her return to work. A number of studies have shown how immediate treatment and confidential hospitalization of suicidal physicians can be lifesaving, perhaps even more so than in nonphysician populations, because of physicians' success rates in killing themselves. Sadly, the threats raised by this approach such as a loss of respect in the community or the fear of temporary withdrawal from practice or of a lack of confidentiality and privacy in treatment may be major impediments, stopping physicians from reaching out in a time of crisis and seeking effective treatment.

For Dr. Johar and Dr. Turner, then, there are three issues to work through over the first few months of therapy: a safety plan, an agreed-on long-term treatment program, and an approach to resolve the loss of sense of self-identity that occurs whenever a patient, especially a physician, is diagnosed with a major mental illness.

The first issue to address, as Dr. Johar requested, is the need for a formalized intervention plan to be put in place if it looks like she is becoming suicidal or psychotic. As discussed in Chapter 1, female physicians have a substantially higher (2.5–4 times higher) rate of completed suicide than age-matched nonphysician females because they use more lethal means (Andrew 2017), even though they actually attempt suicide less frequently. Consequently, any female physician, such as Dr. Johar, has to be taken even more seriously than the average patient if she feels suicidal. A safety plan is of even greater importance for female physicians than it would be for age-matched female nonphysicians, and all physicians treating female doctors need to be very aware of this gender risk paradox.

The safety plan has to include a process that will get the physician patient to be psychiatrically assessed even if she does not herself want this to happen. Usually the plan, which may well be in the form of a written signed contract, will involve the patient's partner and a series of trusted friends and colleagues who know about the individual's illness and who have specifically agreed to monitor the individual and to take specific actions. These may include informing the patient's treating physician or team if they are concerned about the person, or even taking the individual to the emergency department. With physicians, for many of whom remaining in control is a major psychological issue, creating such a plan can be challenging but essential, and it's quite rightly an early goal of Dr. Johar's therapy with Dr. Turner.

A second, related goal is for Dr. Johar to learn more about her illness, to discuss this in detail with Dr. Turner, and to be able to make informed decisions about the best available treatment choices for herself. Most patients with bipolar disorders can ultimately manage their treatment, to a great extent, by themselves, but this process does take time and effort, as well as often quite a lot of adjustments in terms of working out the best medication, lifestyle, support, and therapy regimens. For physicians the stakes are higher than for many other patients because of the absolute importance of keeping themselves healthy in order to be able to continue to practice well and ensure patient safety. Adherence to a biopsychosocial treatment plan is the first rule, and in Dr. Johar's case, it is clear that this has been a problem in the past, given that she had two psychotic episodes in 3 months and stopped her medication in between. In her setting the extra structure of having a contract with her hospital well-being committee to ensure she is adherent with her medication and therapy regimen, as discussed in more detail in Chapter 9, seems sensible. This extra level of monitoring—including, importantly, the addition of a workplace monitor appointed by the well-being committee, which would be hard for Dr. Turner, as an outside psychiatrist, to arrange—has been shown to help physicians keep themselves well. After a few years, and with proof that Dr. Johar is able to adhere to her own treatment appropriately, the hospital committee contract would cease.

The third major issue for Dr. Turner to focus on is Dr. Johar's loss of sense of self and how Dr. Turner can help her work through the issue of her being a physician who has a bipolar disorder—to accept that she is not as fit or healthy as she would like to be, and that she is not perfect, as physicians tend to present themselves to their patients. The aim is to allow Dr. Johar to resolve the internal feelings of loss and distress that inevitably occur, and move forward, able to manage her illness, while not feeling too stigmatized or ashamed. Individual therapy with Dr. Turner would be very helpful here, but so too would be attendance at a physician or health professional support group, where Dr. Johar can discuss her feelings and sense of loss with other healthcare providers who have gone through, or are going through, similar episodes of emotional loss and distress. Such groups are widely available in most major cities and are certainly something that Dr. Turner should discuss with her patient in future sessions.

The next major issue of importance after the three immediate ones just discussed is the wide range of special issues that affect female physicians, especially female academic physicians such as Dr. Johar, and, more specifically, how they can cope with the joint role expectations of being a professional as well as a wife and parent. This is especially important in medicine, where about half of all medical students are now female, and will become more important in future, especially in medical specialties such as primary care and psychiatry, in which there are already significant shortages of physicians. Work-life balance and sharing responsibilities at home more fairly should be part of discussions with male and female physicians. Dr. Johar focused on the solution for her as being the need to increase her resiliency, which is indubitably true and important, but resiliency is only part of the answer, and there may need to be much larger changes to the whole culture, training, and practice of medicine, as discussed in Chapter 10, and the role of physician spouses and families, to really overcome this problem.

An important topic for Dr. Johar and Dr. Turner to address is the daily burden of what some people refer to as being in the role of a "doctor mom." Much has been written about the additional weight that this places on many female physicians that is not usually present for males, as women have been traditionally responsible for most "domestic" responsibilities, which makes achieving a work-life balance more challenging. It is helpful to have support systems in place, such as reliable childcare and regular household help. Physicians who work long hours both professionally and at home are at risk for burnout from one or both environments.

At a professional career level it's now widely accepted that women academics like Dr. Johar have another level of stress on top of the stress experienced by female physicians whose work is primarily patient focused. The need for academics to combine teaching and research with clinical work, while advancing into administrative leadership roles, requires more mentoring and coaching to support professional advancement. The Association of American Medical Colleges (2014) produced an important review regarding the state of women in academic medicine, noting that the pipeline of women in academic medicine gradually narrows, with 47% of matriculants from medical school being female, 38% being faculty, 21% being full professors, and 16% being deans. Women also show clear preferences for certain specialties, with 83% of residents in OB/GYN being female, 71% in pediatrics, 55% in family medicine and psychiatry, and 54% in pathology, and relatively small numbers in most of the surgical specialties. The AAMC has documented the extra financial, coaching, and mentoring needs of academic women required to enable them to overcome this pipeline effect, and to broaden to other specialties, and has strongly recommended that medical schools increase resources for these activities and encourage the development of "Women in Medicine" groups, as Dr. Johar described. Women academics report their major needs to succeed as being clear expectations about the role and path of advancement, an equitable and diverse workplace and access to opportunities for development and advancement (AAMC 2014), and these are all areas that Dr. Johar needs to take up with her departmental chair and her colleagues to help her own advancement.

Finally, a remarkably large number of physicians from other countries are attracted to the United States to train and possibly live permanently in this country. They come from many differing backgrounds and cultures and for countless different reasons. They may be refugees from war-torn countries like Syria or Iraq, both of which have proud traditions of excellent medical training and practice, or they may come by choice, attracted by graduate training or academic opportunities in American centers of excellence. They may or may not speak fluent English. Many do not end up being able to work as physicians in the United States because they cannot pass the step examinations that all students have to take and, therefore, cannot obtain a place in a residency program. Looking at Dr. Johar's past history, it's evident that she should have been treated for depression years before her recent psychotic breaks. She may have been left undiagnosed, and struggling, both because of the culture she came from, where mental illness is highly stigmatized, as she described to Dr. Turner, and its treatment is not seen from a medical perspective as a high-prestige endeavor, and because of the relative lack of preparedness of medical colleagues to identify illnesses in each other, as discussed in Chapter 2.

Kirmayer et al. (2011) have reviewed the types of mental health problems that generally affect immigrants and have commented on what has been called the "healthy immigrant effect," whereby the overall mental health of immigrants tends initially to be better than that of the general population in both sending and receiving countries. This reflects the reality that immigrants have to pass through a number of filters to achieve immigrant status, which in Dr. Johar's case meant doing extra medical exams and residency training to be able to work in the United States. Over time, though, the level of immigrant mental health, in those who have volunteered to move to a different country and are not refugees who have been forced to relocate, tends to worsen and typically ends up matching the level of the receiving general population. Dr. Johar had a fairly sheltered upbringing in India, and while she likely had a genetic vulnerability to bipolar disorder, her illness did not declare itself until she had her first child, which is fairly common among patients with bipolar disorder in general. It is likely that her cultural background, with her perfectionistic drive for success and consequent fear of failure, as well as her internal determination to succeed, made her less likely to seek treatment initially, leading her to struggle on through her residency untreated, but that her gradual acculturation within the United States led her to be more accepting of treatment later in life.

It is hoped that after several years of recurrent mood swings, Dr. Johar has finally found a physician who treats her appropriately by explicitly communicating with her to ensure physician-patient boundaries are maintained, who does not assume the existence of extra knowledge beyond that of an intelligent nonphysician patient, and who takes her sociocultural background and academic ambitions fully into account. The task for Dr. Johar is to gradually accommodate to the idea that she, as a physician, is also going to be a long-term patient and that she has a serious lifelong disease that requires constant management and adherence to a treatment and monitoring plan.

References

Andrew LB: Physician suicide. Medscape, June 12, 2017. Available at: http://emedicine.medscape.com/article/806779-overview. Accessed January 28, 2018.

Alfandre D, Clever S, Farber NJ, et al: Caring for "very important patients"—ethical dilemmas and suggestions for practical management. Am J Med 129(2):143–147, 2016 26522793

Association of American Medical Colleges: The state of women in academic medicine. 2014. Available at: https://members.aamc.org/eweb/upload/The%20State%20of%20Women%20in%20Academic%20Medicine%202013-2014%20FINAL.pdf. Accessed January 28, 2018.

Kirmayer LJ, Narasiah L, Munoz M, et al; Canadian Collaboration for Immigrant and Refugee Health (CCIRH): Common mental health problems in immigrants and refugees: general approach in primary care. CMAJ 183(12):E959–E967, 2011 20603342

National Institute of Mental Health: Bipolar disorder in adults. 2017. Available at: https://www.nimh.nih.gov/health/statistics/prevalence/bipolar-disorder-among-adults.shtml. Accessed January 28, 2018.

Yellowlees PM, Shore JH: Telepsychiatry and Health Technologies: A Guide for Mental Health Professionals. Arlington, VA, American Psychiatric Association Publishing, 2018

Caring for the Carers

DR. ANDREW BROWN'S CELL PHONE RANG, showing him that Dr. Melissa Burt, the chair of surgery, was on the line.

"Hi, Andrew, I hope all is well with you. Have you got a few minutes to discuss one of my surgeons that I believe the Well-Being Committee should review?"

"Certainly. I think I know who we may be going to talk about. Mark in Medical Administration phoned to give me a broad overview earlier today and told me to expect a call from you. I assume this is about the on-call surgeon last night who smelled of alcohol and was taken off service after being reported by the nursing staff."

"I'm afraid that's right. I came in myself urgently to see him about 10 P.M. last night and had to relieve him of his duties. He had certainly been drinking and smelled of alcohol, and was very angry and hostile towards me, especially when I phoned Mark who, as chief medical officer, insisted that he have a blood alcohol done STAT."

"Did you have much of a discussion with him last night and find out what was going on?"

"No, he was really not in the mood for that. I told him I would see him this morning and have just finished a long painful meeting with him. He seemed a bit more contrite, up to when I told him I was putting him on administrative leave until you and your committee have had a chance to assess him. I think he thought he could just apologize and that all would be forgotten."

Andrew Brown, a kindly looking psychiatrist in his fifties wearing a somewhat worn brown jacket over a well-pressed white shirt and an expensive-looking light blue silk tie, looked out of his clinic window as he listened to his colleague. He raised his hand to sweep his long, rather disheveled gray hair backward while mentally calculating when he might be able to see this surgeon urgently and how he might rearrange his already busy schedule to do this.

"Was this a surprise last night, or is there some background of significance that I should know?" he responded.

"You won't be surprised to hear that there is. Dr. Sandford is a full professor and well known for his research in lower GI surgical techniques. He has always been a difficult and rather irritable man, but he specializes in surgery for patients who have Crohn's disease or ulcerative colitis, and as you know they can be very complicated chronically ill individuals both surgically and medically, so he does have a stressful job, without doubt. I think we have just gotten used to his frustrating irritability over the years, but I've received more and more complaints from his patients in recent months, and also from several colleagues, and have actually spoken to him on two occasions about this. On both occasions he flatly denied that there were any problems and blamed everything on the people who complained about him. Even today he was mainly angry with the nursing staff. He continued to deny any alcohol problems and just seemed to want to bluster his way through the interview with me. However, I am assuming alcohol is the issue, especially with his blood alcohol of 0.09 last night, taken several hours after he would have last had a drink. There is no doubt that he would have been operating in an intoxicated state if he hadn't been reported. When do you think you could see him?"

"I can clear some time at 5 P.M. tonight after clinic and could see him then as long as I can find another member of the Well-Being Committee to see him with me. We always have two of us do any assessments, both to help each other clinically and to protect ourselves against any complaints. Can you give him my details and ask him to email me to confirm that time, while I chase up a committee member urgently?"

Later that day Dr. Sandford met with Dr. Brown and Dr. Post, a neurologist who had been available at short notice. Dr. Sandford, a short, somewhat overweight, balding bespectacled man with a graying moustache who was wearing a white lab coat over rather scruffy crumpled pants and shirt, started speaking immediately, not giving Dr. Brown or Dr. Post the remotest opportunity to direct the initial conversation.

"I can't believe I am here seeing you people. This is so humiliating and so very unfair. I've put in 10 years at this hospital working long shifts despite days of extreme exhaustion with patients who constantly want more and more from me. I haven't taken a vacation in the last 3 years just so I can keep up with the workload. So this is the thanks I get from the so-called leadership of this hospital. I feel like I'm being called to the principal's office. My chair doesn't know how hard I've been working, and it's been really hard dealing with other staff who don't appreciate me either. If we could just get some regular staffing in the clinic and the OR so that I can train them on how I want everything done, all would be OK. Then they accuse me of drinking when I'm on call. Of course, I do that sometimes. I'm on call for my own patients almost all the time. If they're in crisis, I can't let someone else operate on them, because this is very difficult surgery and no one else does it as well as me. And then I have to do the routine hospital calls at least two nights per week on top of that. So what if I have a drink or two to relax at home on my own time? How dare that OR tech report me for a little alcohol on my breath? And then he gets the charge nurse to get on my back too. They grossly exaggerated the situation, and finally Dr. Burt felt she needed to come in from home. They should have all just left me alone to get on with my operating. I don't know how the blood alcohol came back so high. Obviously a lab error. I'm going to have that investigated. I have had big concerns about our lab work for a long time now, and this is just another example of their incompetence."

Finally Dr. Brown managed to get a word in.

"Dr. Sandford, do you know why we have asked you here?"

"Of course I do. A ridiculous allegation was made about me in error last night, and it's all being blown out of proportion now. There is nothing wrong with me. I know what you two are going to accuse me of, but it won't work. I'm not an alcoholic. I don't have a problem. I'm a busy surgeon and I have things to do tonight. I need to finish this meeting and be out of here as quickly as possible. Just ask your questions and let's be done with this."

The meeting continued in the same vein for another hour, and later that night Dr. Sandford recounted his version of it to his long-suffering wife.

"I told them I wasn't going to even answer their stupid questions other than to say 'no.' Nothing more. This was their show. There were a lot of long pauses while my two 'colleagues' looked at each other. That's when my trial began. They launched into an attack on me. At least that's what it felt like to me. They tried to portray themselves not only as the patient support team but as mine too. They spoke about the purpose of the Well-Being Committee and why I was brought in to meet with them and tried to convince me that they were there to help me, all the while confronting me with lots of innuendo. Then they brought out a long list of concerns from several physicians and other staff that had come to them via my chair, who seems to have already sent them a whole series of written complaints. I began to feel very uncomfortable and nervous. I got quite sweaty and anxious. It was all so unfair. Then it got worse. They brought up several patients and their families who had complained about the way I spoke with them. They used words like 'condescending,' 'demeaning,' and 'rude.' My heart sank and I wanted to run out the door. There were too many complaints. How could this be?"

He continued. "They said this was a first meeting, but it went on for almost 2 hours. I was exhausted. At the end they said they thought I was an alcoholic, which is nonsense. The choices they offered were beyond painful. I could either leave and face administrative action from my chair, or I have to sign a contract to deal with what they described as my alcohol problem. They also required that I be seen by an outside psychiatrist to be evaluated and treated. What they suggested all seemed so extreme and unnecessary, but I had no choice. I couldn't walk out on my job and my career. I can't believe the consequence of just having a couple of drinks when on call."

"What's going to happen next?" asked his wife.

"From what they said it seems they're going to collect some more information about me and discuss me at their committee meeting and then come back to me with some final recommendations. In the meantime, they told me I have to stop drinking completely, which I have done lots of times before as you know. They're going to send me some details of how I can start being monitored with regular random breath analyses, which I guess I have no choice but to start. The results of all of these will be sent to my psychiatrist, and she'll contact Dr. Brown if any are positive. They also talked about individual and group therapy and maybe going to Alcoholics Anonymous, but I really pushed back on that. I'll just prove to them that I can keep sober, and then we should be able to finish all this."

A week later the hospital Well-Being Committee assembled for its first meeting of the year.

Dr. Brown, the committee chair for several years, addressed his 15 colleagues and 2 administrative staff who were present for the committee meeting.

"As this is the first meeting of the year, I wish to briefly address a few issues as a reminder for all of us, and for our three new members, to ensure we are all on the same page. Please do all review the committee Web site, where you'll find all the bylaws and policies and procedures that relate to us. I'd like to particularly note that we have several aims as a group and are a very focused committee with a specific set of roles to play."

He looked around the table, observing his colleagues carefully from behind his rimless glasses. This was his ninth year as chair of this committee, and he was proud of the work they did.

"Firstly, we are a committee mandated by the Joint Commission to ensure patient and health system quality, and we're here to promote the general physical and mental well-being of all members of our medical staff. It's important that you remember that we are not a punitive group and are never involved in making disciplinary orders against our medical staff. We're available to help all staff receive treatment if they wish to be helped, but if they have some medical or psychiatric problems that are impairing their practice and do not want our assistance, then they will be dealt with through the usual health system administrative channels." He stopped talking for a moment to emphasize this issue, and then continued his introduction.

"As a committee we have offered a voluntary screening program for our medical staff for health problems that might impair their practice for a number of years, but we also try to improve their health by supporting their practice needs and preventing problems. As such a major role of the committee is to spend time educating our physicians and especially our leadership and other staff about the importance of physician health. After all, if your physicians are not healthy, how are they going to help their patients effectively? With respect to this role as a committee, we focus on four main areas of illness or disorder that can adversely affect our physicians' capacity to practice. These are the potential presence of psychiatric disorders, including suicidal ideation, substance misuse and addictions, and neurocognitive disorders such as memory problems, especially related to brain diseases and the aging process. In recent years we have also engaged in a fourth area with what we call 'disruptive physicians,' or those colleagues who we believe have severe personality disorders, who tend to be arrogant and hard to get along with, and who have an adverse impact mainly on their colleagues and on the internal processes and workflows of the health system."

He continued: "Of course, the final part of our work is what everyone knows we do, and we tend to do this in the second half of each meeting.

This involves reviewing and assessing any colleagues referred to the committee and, if necessary, arranging treatment and monitoring for them for any of the illnesses or behavioral disorders that they have. Any questions or comments?"

Dr. Martin, an OB/GYN and a new member of the committee, spoke up. "Thank you for including me in this committee. I'm very interested in it and would like to help do some of the assessments of individuals referred to the committee if possible. What I don't understand is how physicians get referred to us. What is the usual process?"

"There are lots of differing ways," Dr. Brown responded. "But most people come via a colleague or senior medical educator or administrator. So for faculty it is frequently the chair of a department or division who will phone or email me, as the usual first point of contact, as happened with a new referral we saw last week. Referring educators and administrators have often had a number of meetings with the person they are referring and commonly phone one of us for advice even before they discuss suggesting a referral to the individual. In fact, I find that I can often give helpful advice to them at that stage that allows them to handle the situation without sending the physician to us."

"What about suicides, or suicidal behavior? How often does that come up as a concern?" asked a surgeon who had been on the committee for several years. "It seems to be a common topic when I listen to the cases we discuss in this meeting, but how common do you think it is?"

"That's an interesting question that I probably should know the answer to. As you all know, probably at least 400 physicians per year, in numbers equal across genders, do tragically die by suicide. Fortunately, we have not had any physician suicides that I know of in the 8 years I have been chairing this committee, and I hope we remain that way. As you correctly say, though, we do have several physicians each year who are actively suicidal and for whom we have to intervene and arrange treatment urgently. I would guess that about half of those come via the screening program we run, which specifically identifies active suicidal ideation, and half from referrals from colleagues. Obviously, we see those people urgently, and one of the psychiatrists on the committee is always involved in those situations."

Marjorie Halston, a senior administrator who had been on the committee longer than Dr. Brown, commented, "I think you're right. Having worked at the health system for 25 years, I can't recall a suicide of a physician while they were here, although we do know of three that I remember who died by suicide within a few years of leaving here. This was all over 15 years ago before we had this committee, but in two of the cases medical administration knew the physicians had problems while they were here, and unfortunately they both turned out to be addicts, one involving alcohol and the other narcotics. At that time we weren't nearly so ready to intervene and help as we are now, and I've always regretted that we didn't do more for them. I think our lack of suicides is mainly just that we have been lucky though. There have been several local physician suicides that have really affected the medical community that some of you will know about. One was a medical student who killed himself by jumping off the top of the medical school a few years ago, and of course the private health system across town had that awful tragic run of two physicians who killed themselves within a few months about 5 years ago."

"Thanks indeed, Marjorie. I really appreciate your depth of knowledge about both our system and the other medical communities in the city," said Dr. Brown. "I think we have had enough of an introductory discussion, so let's turn to the agenda."

After all members of the committee nodded their assent, Dr. Brown continued. "As usual, the first item on the agenda is a short wellness activity that Dr. Newark, from Emergency Medicine, has volunteered to lead this year. For those who are new to the committee, we literally try to not just talk the talk, but also walk the walk, so we almost always start these meetings with a 5-minute wellness activity that can be anything from meditation to yoga, tai chi, stretching, or mindfulness. We greatly value creativity and experiment with as wide a range of simple, easy activities as possible—especially ones that we might be able to use ourselves when we are in stressful situations."

Dr. Newark, a fit-looking man in his forties wearing scrubs, took over and, much to the surprise of the new members, led the committee through a 5-minute mindfulness eating exercise that involved everyone eating several raisins very slowly and thoughtfully, so that they fully experienced the taste, feel, and texture of the fruit, while relaxing and focusing on their inner thoughts, reactions, and sensations in silence. Although several members thought that the exercise seemed silly initially, it actually turned out to be effective. People slowed down and became less distracted and more engaged.

Dr. Brown then moved on to the rest of the agenda, the first half of which focused on well-being activities that the committee was involved in that were primarily meant to ultimately influence organizational change within the health system. The first item was a report on a conference on burnout that two of the committee members had been to recently, which led on to a discussion about whether the committee should be proposing a survey on the level of burnout in the health system physicians or not. There was little consensus on this. Most committee members took the view that any survey would simply show that up to 40% of respondents had some symptoms of burnout, as had been shown in numerous other health systems surveyed, and that it was pointless doing such a survey unless there were some major interventions planned, in which case there could be surveys done both before and after the intervention. This was followed by a report on the number of physicians who had participated in the anonymous online depression and suicide screening program in the past year, and how many had been referred for treatment. Several committee members commented that the screening program seemed well established and that they had heard very positive comments about it from their own departmental chairs. This section of the agenda finished with a discussion on the child-care needs of the health system and how these were perceived as being inadequate. A number of committee members spoke passionately about this issue, giving several examples of young female faculty who were being stretched excessively by the combination of their own child-care demands and their work commitments.

Dr. Brown now moved on to the final part of the agenda, announcing that there were two cases to be discussed, one new referral, Dr. Sandford, and one 6-monthly review of an individual who was on a 3-year behavioral contract for disruptive behavior. Dr. Brown asked Dr. Post to summarize Dr. Sandford's background and presentation for the committee, and then he provided an overview of the assessment and proposed monitoring plan.

"The bottom line, with this surgeon, is that he is in tremendous denial about his long-standing alcohol abuse. He doesn't seem to be physically dependent on alcohol, and he has a history of being able to stop drinking successfully for a month at a time, which he has done on many occasions, but he then relapses and certainly drinks in a fashion that is likely to lead to impaired medical practice. He's also rather depressed and irritable and needs a combination of treatment for that and his alcohol problem, possibly even a 12-step outpatient program and medication-assisted treatment. So I think given his lack of insight and denial, he certainly needs a monitoring program and at least a 3-year contract with us."

Dr. Brown turned to the committee for their comments and was pleased at their level of agreement with the plan, which they agreed to implement.

Dr. Brown continued, looking down at the agenda sheet. "Now let's move on to the next review. This is an individual who has been doing very well and who we have been monitoring for about 3 years now. Dr. Garden and I saw him originally. Perhaps you could summarize his situation for everyone, please, Dr. Garden?"

Dr. Garden, a bespectacled, rather intense-looking anesthesiologist in his fifties, wearing a white lab coat over his scrubs, sat forward and spoke quietly. "As you all know, this individual that we have been monitoring is a very highly respected senior professor in a surgical specialty whom I work with in surgery on occasions and who has a long history of narcotic abuse. He and I know each other well and have ended up going to some of the same groups for health professionals with addiction problems. He has come to me on several occasions for advice and support, given that I have over 20 years of sobriety from alcohol. As you have all heard at prior meetings of this committee, he seems to have really embraced his recovery, having done the full 12-step program and attended the 6-week outpatient day program we insisted on as part of his contract, as well as following up with the groups, individual counseling, and, of course, random body fluid monitoring. Despite this he really worries me. He is asking if we can stop monitoring him and cancel his contract sometime soon, but he really doesn't have a good reason for this. He says it is all too much trouble and he doesn't want to take up our time when we have others to look after, and tells me he intends to continue with his pathway of sobriety. I have discussed the treatment outcomes with him and have made it clear that the only studies we have are of 5 years of follow-up, at which stage he has an 80% chance of remaining sober and continuing to be fully licensed according to the figures. I've used myself as an example and how I've had to continue the sobriety struggle literally every day. Despite this he wants the committee to consider dropping the monitoring contract, and he asked me to propose this to all of you. His final argument is that he's now traveling so much more than he used to with the success of his research that he finds the monitoring process less easy to fit in, and he is worried about his narcotic abuse being found out at a time that his career has really blossomed."

"Interesting. And knowing him, I am not completely surprised," said Dr. Brown. "Comments, anyone?"

A surgeon committee member commented. "He's someone who has been very successful in the past at hiding his illness. Let's not forget that he probably went at least a decade likely operating on many occasions in an at least partially inebriated state, especially when on call. I see this as another attempt by him to deny his disease. It's rather ironic that he seems to want to put himself at risk just when his career is really taking off in a big way."

Dr. Brown interceded. "We're going to have to finish the meeting soon, and I want to be respectful of all of your schedules and not keep you late. He seems to be doing very well overall, and we don't want to put him at any extra risk of relapse, but I personally don't really have a good understanding of why he is so keen to stop his contract at this stage and would like to know more about that, as well as have the chance to discuss the latest research outcomes with him. Perhaps the best thing for us to do is to have Dr. Garden and me meet with him again and review his whole situation. We'll then bring our recommendation back to the committee for you all to review. Is that a reasonable compromise?"

The members of the committee generally nodded assent, and several got up from their chairs, starting to move toward the door.

"Thanks to all of you for coming. I look forward to seeing you next month," Dr. Brown said, as the room emptied rapidly.

Three weeks later Dr. Brown met once again with Dr. Sandford to give him feedback from the Well-Being Committee and to arrange his monitoring contract.

Dr. Sandford was much less defensive than previously and started the conversation by saying, "My initial session with the psychiatrist went better than I had expected. It seemed like most of the time was spent with me just talking with him. He didn't say much, and somehow I began to unload about how unfair the Well-Being Committee had been to me. I let him know I did not have a drinking problem and that the lab messed up the results twice. Despite this he set up the random urine tests, and I know you're insisting on a work site monitor for the next 3 years. You know I still feel like I have no choice, but I decided all I can do is to prove you and the psychiatrist to be all wrong."

A few months later, in a reflective mood, Dr. Sandford was talking to his wife one evening. "This has been much harder than I expected. I have been really craving drinks, and in the end asked my psychiatrist to put me on medication to reduce my cravings, and to my surprise it has made quite a big difference. I hate to admit it but I think I might have been wrong. I've begun to wonder if I actually did have a drinking problem. It was much harder to stop the evening martinis than I thought, even though you have been great and have joined me in giving them up. I was surprised at how I couldn't get to sleep for weeks when I first stopped drinking and I didn't feel right in the first few months. I can see I would not have done this without the support and monitoring I've had. I had no choice. I couldn't lose my job. I had to get through this even if it meant cooperating with the Well-Being Committee. So I did. And to my surprise I've had some really positive comments from the nurses at work, and even from some patients. I must have been more irritable than I thought."

"What else do you think has helped you?" Mrs. Sandford asked.

"I saw the psychiatrist a lot in the beginning, and he helped me become aware of how out of balance my life had become. I had become used to working to fill my days and drinking to sort of make me numb. I know I was ignoring you and the children. I was lonely and bored with my life. I withdrew and wasn't doing anything with you, or with the friends I used to have. I had no one to play golf with or even meet for coffee. No one at all. I used to love golf but I haven't played in years. I needed help to turn things around and see how different I was. The psychiatrist was surprisingly confrontational in a gentle way on these issues, and I have learned to really respect and trust him."

He continued. "We're talking more about my alcohol problems now, and how I was more dependent on it than I ever admitted. I actually find the random urine tests quite helpful now. I know I can't cheat, and they're a sort of safety structure that keeps me on the straight and narrow, even though I have several more years of them. Oddly enough they're part of my healing. I know that now. I know why they have a Well-being Committee and why they follow up and monitor physicians like me. I think they really did save my career. I was never punished for what I did, and luckily I didn't harm any patients. It seems weird to admit it, but I'm actually grateful people at work had the courage to report me before it was too late, and my psychiatrist is encouraging me to talk to the nurses who reported me to thank them. Maybe I'll have the strength to do that one day."

Commentary

This chapter is primarily about the response of health care organizations and institutions to the issue of physician health and well-being, and the impact that well-organized physician well-being committees, taking on the function of a physician health program, can have on individual physicians.

Physician well-being committees vary greatly in scope and practice around the country, primarily depending on whether they are in a state without a centralized physician health program (PHP), such as California, Nebraska, or Wisconsin, or whether such a program exists. Theoretically all such committees are meant to meet a mandate from the Joint Commission, the national body that accredits health care institutions as discussed below. This scenario is modeled on an idealized medical staff well-being committee currently running in California, where there is no centralized statewide PHP. Health system or hospital well-being committees in California, therefore, have the dual roles, as shown in the scenario, of both supporting physician wellness and assessing and monitoring the treatment of a few internal physicians to ensure patient safety. Examples of such programs are detailed online at the medical staff Web sites from UC

Davis (www.ucdmc.ucdavis.edu/medstaffwellbeing/), Kaiser Permanente (https://scpmgphysicianwellness.kaiserpermanente.org/physician-well-being; Southern California Permanente Medical Group [Kaiser] Medical Staff Well-Being Committee 2014), Stanford Health Care (https://stanfordhealthcare.org/health-care-professionals/medical-staff/leadership-and-medical-staff-committees/medical-staff-committees.html), and other institutions.

The California statewide PHP was closed in 2010 following concerns about its outcomes and practices, and since that time the many health systems in California have had to provide the assessment and monitoring functions of physicians themselves through their physician well-being committees. Contemporaneously an attempt is being made, headed by the California Medical Association (CMA), to re-create and fund an independent statewide PHP. So while the scenario presented in this chapter is not typical of what happens in most U.S. states, it is helpful as an example of how physicians can be helped at a local level, rather than by a single statewide program, which in a state like California, with a population of more than 100,000 physicians, is hard to arrange. The scenario shows both of the major functions required to support and maintain physician health and well-being and demonstrates how this model could work nationally, especially in states where statewide PHPs have attracted substantial criticism or are ineffective. PHPs in most states are primarily responsible for the assessment and monitoring function, which occurs at a statewide level and which, unfortunately, has led, as an unintended consequence, to minimal work being done on physician well-being in most healthcare institutions nationally at the local clinic or hospital level, despite the Joint Commission mandates discussed below.

Statewide PHPs assess and monitor the physicians referred to them, and generally physicians who comply with their recommendations continue to work, provided they are monitored by the PHP, a process that may include regular reports from treating physicians and random drug testing. Statewide PHPs are run in very differing ways, some by independent nonprofit corporations and others by state medical societies, or with the support from state medical boards. They are represented by a national association, the Federation of State Physician Health Programs (FSPHP), which states its four basic principles very clearly on its Web site (Federation of State Physician Health Programs 2018):

> 1) The FSPHP supports the early detection, evaluation and treatment of physicians and other licensed healthcare professionals suffering from addictive, psychiatric, medical, behavioral or other potentially impairing conditions. Appropriate evaluation and treatment of these physicians at

programs experienced with the treatment of professionals in safety sensitive employment will ultimately enhance the health of the provider and better protect the public.

2) The FSPHP strongly opposes discrimination of a physician during licensing, credentialing or at any time, based on a history of addictive, psychiatric, or other illness.

3) The FSPHP supports the use of PHP services, whenever possible, in lieu of disciplinary action. When PHP services are not used, it is less likely that physicians will receive early intervention and appropriate treatment. It is well-known that illness often predates impairment by a period of years. The FSPHP believes earlier intervention in potentially impairing illness to be more efficacious than intervention in later stages of disease.

4) The FSPHP believes privacy and confidentiality of a physician's health and treatment history must be paramount in the relationships between PHPs and ill physicians or other licensed healthcare professionals to allow those in need of help to come forward without fear of punishment, disciplinary action, embarrassment, or professional isolation. Confidentiality enhances the opportunity for recovery, and incentive to participate in early intervention.

These principles are very important and explain why PHPs are often known as "diversion" programs, because they're programs that are highly confidential and allow physicians with addictions or psychiatric problems to continue working while they receive monitored treatment. This is exactly what is described in the case scenario and, as long as physicians are practicing in a manner that is unimpaired, is the best outcome possible and a process that should be strongly supported.

PHPs have come under significant criticism by some consumer groups, who argue that doctors should be treated openly like everyone else and should not have access to a secret treatment process that ultimately ensures that patients can't find out if a doctor is being treated for a specific disorder that might impair his or her practice. It's true that PHPs don't work in a consistent manner and that their scope of services varies, with most focusing on assessing and monitoring physicians with psychiatric or substance-related problems rather than on the prevention of illness and promotion of physician well-being. Several PHPs have attracted strong criticism, accused of being, on the one hand, programs where doctors protect their own at the expense of patients or, on the other, programs that are overly coercive and poorly overseen and audited. Some are under fire currently and may be terminated. Anderson (2015) has written a balanced summary of these issues, noting the intrusion of legal opinions and the expense of some programs to the referred physicians as important negative issues stopping physicians from either referring themselves voluntarily or, once referred, obtaining appropriate care. A number of these PHPs are well recognized as being leading-edge organizations nationally, however, providing excellent care for large numbers of physicians and generally helping to educate the medical profession on the importance of physician health and well-being. The Colorado PHP (https://cphp.org) and Massachusetts PHP (http://www.massmed.org/phshome) are examples of such programs and also have comprehensive, informative Web sites, with both now receiving 40%–60% of their physician referrals as self-referrals, indicating that they've gained very substantial levels of trust and respect within the state physician community, a process that typically takes many years.

One of the most problematic areas for any PHP or well-being committee is its relationship with the physician regulator in each state, the state medical board. Many physicians do not realize that the medical board, which licenses them, is actually a consumer protection organization. The medical board is not primarily an organization that is designed to help doctors. Its primary aims are to license physicians and to protect the public. Doctors who are reported to the medical board are sometimes surprised when they find out that the board can be quite punitive and will tend to philosophically take the side of public protection rather than trying to assist the doctor in its decision making. The bulk of every medical board budget is spent on enforcement, not licensing, and for this reason a primary aim of any PHP or well-being committee is to detect and treat physicians early in their illness or disorder, prior to their developing any practice impairment, and hence avoid the requirement to report to the medical board. Reporting of any physician who is impaired and has his or her credentialing or scope of practice changed because of an illness is required by most state medical boards, all of which differ in their legal definitions and timelines. Having said this, the leaders of most PHPs and well-being committees try hard to have good relationships with their local medical boards in order to be able to work together as much as possible, bearing in mind their sometimes rather different objectives.

The CMA has published an excellent set of guidelines for physician well-being committees (California Medical Association 2015) that may be read in parallel with a guideline for selecting physician health services published by California Public Protection & Physician Health (2010). The CMA guideline notes that an "individual health" or well-being function is mandated by the Joint Commission (2001), the national group that accredits hospitals, to support the personal health and facilitate rehabilitation of medical staff through "a process to identify and manage matters of individual health for licensed independent practitioners which is separate from actions taken for disciplinary purposes." The Joint Commission process must include all of the following nine elements:

1. Education of practitioners and other organizational staff about illness and impairment recognition issues
2. Self-referral by a practitioner
3. Referral by others and maintaining informant confidentiality
4. Referral of the practitioner to the appropriate professional internal or external resources for evaluation, diagnosis, and treatment of the condition or concern
5. Maintenance of the confidentiality of the practitioner seeking referral or referred for assistance, except as limited by law or ethical obligation or when the health and safety of a patient is threatened
6. Evaluation of the credibility of a complaint, allegation, or concern
7. Monitoring of the practitioner and the safety of patients until the rehabilitation is complete, and periodically thereafter if required
8. Reporting to the organized medical staff leadership instances in which a practitioner is providing unsafe treatment
9. Initiation of appropriate actions when a practitioner fails to complete the required rehabilitation program

Hospitals and community physician associations have a reasonably wide range of flexibility as to how they manage their well-being committees to meet these mandated Joint Commission requirements, and as to the level of scope that they cover, but their primary purpose is to focus on the needs of physicians while at the same time considering patient safety. Committees are specifically advised not to provide treatment to physicians referred to them; instead, it is intended that they monitor treatment provided by others to ensure that the physicians remain well and that patient safety is upheld.

Unfortunately, although the Joint Commission does evaluate this mandated standard, little change seems to have happened in the more than a decade since the standard was introduced. This particular standard does not seem to be viewed as particularly important in most inspections when compared with, for example, the 2017 national patient safety goals, which include better patient identification, improved caregiver communication, safer use of medications, and reduction in the harm associated with clinical alarm systems and healthcare–associated infections, among others. It would seem to be important to reduce physician suicide and improve physician well-being, and perhaps one day we'll see national goals like those in this standard.

In most hospitals and healthcare institutions around the country, the well-being committees are mainly focused on being a referral pathway to send physicians having difficulties on to the local statewide PHPs, and they have little other activity, meeting, if at all, only a few times per year. In states such as California, where the committees need to be much more active, most meet monthly at least and are multidisciplinary in nature, as shown in the scenario. The CMA 2015 guideline (California Medical Association 2015) specifically encourages the inclusion of members from several medical specialties, as well as experts in addiction and psychiatry and "qualified persons recovering from alcoholism or other chemical dependence." Most committees function primarily to assess and monitor colleagues who are referred to them as a result of concerns about their capacity to practice as a result of psychiatric or substance-related concerns. Relatively few such committees historically have involved themselves with physicians who have neurocognitive disorders, or disorders related to aging, or who are disruptive, although this is now gradually changing as the nature and expectations of medical practice and professional behavior are also evolving. In some health systems the wellness and preventive approaches to healthcare described in the scenario are managed by a separate committee entirely, and in others anonymity is not sought or required for those individuals managed by such committees. Indeed, in many committees, physicians who are being monitored might be asked to appear and meet with the whole committee, which of course means that they have no anonymity within the committee itself, although anonymity is maintained to the external world.

As described in the scenario, well-being committees tend to attract physicians who have a specific interest in physician health either because they're interested in the patient care aspects, which is likely the primary motivation for most members who have backgrounds in either psychiatry or addiction medicine, or because they've seen examples in their own practice that have led them to realize the importance of the topic. The chairs of these committees tend to stay in the role for several years for two reasons. First, being chair can be challenging, and it can take several years to become truly confident in dealing with the numerous ethical issues that arise, especially the potential overlap in the role of the committee to monitor, treat, and help, and the needs of the health system to ensure patient safety, and potentially provide corrective administrative actions. There is no substitute for experience in these situations, as the difficulties that affect physicians referred to well-being committees, as described throughout this book, are unpredictable and frequently highly complicated and need to be dealt with using extreme care and sensitivity. Second, there is a need for long-term continuity on the committee, and while most members may serve 2–4 years, as on most hospital committees, the long-term nature of monitoring contracts, usually 3–5 years, and the recurrent nature of some referrals mean that the history of the committee's work and interactions with monitored physicians is of great importance. Here long-term membership from some members is not just helpful but essential. The other unusual "qualification" for the membership of some committee members is their own psychiatric or addiction-related history. In the scenario presented in this chapter, the anesthesiologist on the committee is open about his own alcohol addiction and his daily continuing struggle, and it's not at all uncommon for such individuals, when they are stable and in long-term remission, to be able to perform a valuable task on well-being committees. They are able to empathize well with those physicians being monitored and frequently are able to meet with individuals who are going through the assessment process to reassure them that the committee is really there to help them, and that the process is not punitive and that it's possible to recover from their disease or disorder and come out the other side with their license and professional reputation intact. Similarly, it's not uncommon for some committee members to have developed an interest in this area because they have known physician friends or colleagues who have died by suicide or who have major problems and they hope to learn how to prevent such events recurring for others. Other members of the committee, such as residents, may be there to learn and understand the importance of professionalism, as well as to give as broad an input as possible, while others typically come from disciplines such as emergency medicine or anesthesiology, where there is a high level of need.

There are a number of other issues of importance regarding well-being committees. First, such committees are less easily available to the more than 50% of physicians in the United States who are in small or solo private practices and who do not have any, or many, colleagues who can help advise or refer them if they start having health problems. Physicians who practice in this way are already at risk of becoming isolated and professionally and personally lonely, and without access to supportive colleagues, they're at risk of being even slower or later in seeking out treatment or care for any psychiatric or addiction-related problems they might be developing. This is the reason that the ability to self-refer to PHPs is so important, as described by the Massachusetts and Colorado PHPs, because this gives easier access to this large group of physicians. Even with this capacity, however, physicians in such private practices are at more risk of later referral and assistance than physicians who work in large institutions or group practices, where colleagues can potentially identify ill health or behavioral problems and take action to assist. In states like California, where no central PHP exists, there is literally no place for such private practice physicians to refer themselves, even if they wish to, so it's clear that whether a statewide PHP exists or not, there is also room for other local PHPs or local well-being committees, with the monitoring function illustrated in the scenario. While PHPs and well-being committees are generally consolidating and are now well established in one form or another in every state, it's clear that there needs to be an extension of these programs so that they can be more easily accessible by all physicians, especially those in small private practices. For this to happen, the PHPs in general need to be fully transparent about their scope of services, their costs, and any boundaries and requirements they have on assessment, treatment, and monitoring programs.

Finally, the issue of the health and well-being function of well-being committees is of great importance, but, regrettably, frequently is nonexistent, or only paid lip service to, in most healthcare institutions in most states, with of course some shining exceptions. In the long term the most important function of such committees is to gradually change the culture of healthcare and to make the importance of physician health a key issue. This will happen only slowly and will depend on the interest and commitment of institutional leaders, and how the members of well-being committees can gradually facilitate such change over time. In Chapter 2, I reviewed the work of Shanafelt and Noseworthy (2017) at the Mayo Clinic, including the multiple drivers of burnout in physicians that occur at the individual, work unit, organizational, and national levels. Many of these factors can be addressed within well-being committees, especially the organizational (and attitudinal) ones, and in the scenario in this chapter these include discussions on wellness activities, a screening program, and the need for improved childcare. Other organizational issues that well-being committees can address include improving the electronic medical record system, a continuing major stressor for many physicians as detailed in the cases in Chapters 2 and 10, as well as the use of patient portals, development of appointment systems, opportunities for professional development, the culture of the organization, and the need for physician lounges and private areas for collegial meetings and discussions, among others.

To summarize, the response of the healthcare profession to the fairly recently identified needs of physician health and well-being is still at an early stage. PHPs are well established in most states, and in those places where they do not exist, local well-being committees are taking up much of their role. The outcomes of PHPs, as discussed in Chapter 5, are excellent, although there is relatively little focus on professional education and attitudinal change on this topic. There are still massive gaps in this organizational response, with relatively little impact overall from the Joint Commission–mandated standards, and relatively poor access to care by self-referral for physicians who do not work in large healthcare systems or practice groups. There is more research being done on this broad topic, but there are very few strong research groups beyond the Mayo Clinic and Stanford research teams, and almost no attention being paid to health and impairment issues of physicians in private community practice, an area few research funders prioritize as a focus for funding. There needs to be a much stronger response from organizations and institutions generally than has occurred up to this time, and, it is hoped, such a response will improve over time as the medical profession gradually learns better ways to look after itself while at the same time ensuring that patient care is unimpaired.

References

Anderson PA: Physician health programs: more harm than good? Medscape, August 19, 2015. Available at: https://www.medscape.com/viewarticle/849772#vp_5. Accessed January 29, 2018.

California Medical Association: Physician well-being committees: guidelines. Document no. 5177, January 2015. Available at: https://www.cppph.org/cppph-guidelines/. Accessed January 29, 2018.

California Public Protection and Physician Health: Guidelines for selecting physician health services. May 2010. Available at: https://www.cppph.org/cppph-guidelines/. Accessed January 29, 2018.

Federation of State Physician Health Programs: Frequently asked questions: what are the basic principles of the FSPHP? 2018. Available at: https://www.fsphp.org/about/faqs. Accessed January 29, 2018.

The Joint Commission: Standard MS.11.01.01. January 1, 2001. Available at: http://www.massmed.org/Physician_Health_Services/Joint_Commission/Joint_Commission_Requirement_-_MS_11_01_01/. Accessed January 29, 2018.

Shanafelt TD, Noseworthy JH: Executive leadership and physician well-being: nine organizational strategies to promote engagement and reduce burnout. Mayo Clin Proc 92(1):129–146, 2017 27871627

Southern California Permanente Medical Group (Kaiser) Medical Staff Well-Being Committee: Physician well-being. May 21, 2014. Available at: https://scpmgphysicianwellness.kaiserpermanente.org/physician-well-being. Accessed January 29, 2018.

10

Physician
Heal Thyself

THE EVENING SUN was just setting on yet another beautiful day. Not a cloud in the sky. The fading yellow ball dropped rapidly below the horizon, and bright orange flashes lit the night. Lights and shadows shimmered over the rapidly darkening water as the father and son relaxed in their comfortable white Adirondack chairs, sipping ice tea as they contemplated the sunset together.

Sam, a fit, athletic-looking man in his early thirties, clean-shaven with blond tousled hair, wearing worn board shorts, a shirt adorned with a New York logo, and blue canvas loafers, looked fondly across at his father. He had been looking forward to staying at his dad's seaside unit over this Christmas season and having some one-on-one time with him. Despite this he had a sense of foreboding about how the discussions on the direction of his future medical career would go. He knew his father would raise this topic, and now that the talks were close he rather regretted suggesting that Julie, his fiancée, not come with him to help tell their plans to his dad. He and Julie planned on getting married in a few months, just after they both finished residency, and he was already missing her.

Sam decided that there was no point in waiting for his dad to bring up the topic, so he decided to jump right into the conversation before they started cooking the steaks he had brought.

"Dad, I want to talk to you in some detail about the plans Julie and I have been making for after we're through residency, and I would really like your opinion on what we wish to do. It's amazing what you've done with your life and how influential you've been in not only my choice of going to medical school but then in my following you into emergency medicine. Watching you, and knowing you, has really made me think about my own life, and the decisions I have to make. I know that you've never consciously pushed me in one direction or another and that you've been great in allowing me to make my own decisions, but I'm very aware that you would like me to join your hospital and maybe eventually take over your role as director of the emergency department. We both know you want this, although you've never actually brought it up with me, and that's what I want to discuss with you."

Michael drew his eyes slowly away from the final remnants of the sunset and looked carefully at his only son. He was incredibly proud of him and aware that he must be very careful about what he said and advised his son to do. He was, indeed, hoping Sam would come and work at his hospital. He had always struggled with this wish and truly believed that he had not deliberately tried to excessively influence him in this direction—at least not consciously. But he also realized that he was inevitably an influential figure for Sam.

Michael took a deep breath, taking his time to reply, knowing that they had all evening to continue their conversation over the barbeque that Sam would cook later. He rather wished that he had taken the time to learn how to cook as well as Sam, who always seemed to be learning new cooking skills, and especially how to make interesting barbeque sauces. Where did he find the time for gourmet cooking as a resident? How Michael valued the gift of time, to be able to communicate and share his thoughts and feelings with Sam. He had had no one to open up to since Angie, his ex-wife and Sam's mother, finally left him a decade before, when Sam was in college. He still missed Angie, but he understood that he had really always been married to his work, rather than to her. He no longer blamed her for finding a new husband who was the real life partner she deserved. He tried to think back to his past life and regretted not taking more time off on public holidays like this one where he could have the opportunity of just relaxing and having fun, of getting away from the constant pressure of his medical practice.

Sam looked inquisitively at his father in silence. He admired his father but also felt sorry for him, although he would never tell him this. Sam felt pleased that on some occasions in recent years he had finally succeeded in getting him to put aside his physician persona and to just be his dad. Michael looked somewhat older than his 55 years, and Sam had noted how he had physically slowed down and was no longer able to keep up with his son in waterskiing or beach volleyball. He couldn't help but notice that his dad had put on a few pounds in recent years. Michael had always dressed conservatively, mainly in collared polo shirts even on holidays. This was a sharp contrast to Sam's casual shorts and T-shirts most days. Michael was tall and clean-shaven with heavy bags under both eyes, evidence of many sleep-disturbed nights, with his short wavy gray hair immaculately brushed in the same style that he had worn since he was a teenager. Michael's bifocals were perched on the end of his nose, and Sam felt this gave his father a somewhat aristocratic and intellectual feel. He loved his dad, especially now that he understood all the sacrifices he had made and the hardships he had endured, but he was determined not to emulate his life.

Finally, Michael replied, "Of course I would love you, and also Julie, to come and work at my hospital. As a pair you would be quite a catch for us. It's so difficult for us to recruit physicians nowadays. Having a married couple with such a personal connection to someone like myself would be really welcome. If you want, I can certainly arrange for you to be interviewed for an attending position in the emergency department, although, of course, I can't personally be on the interview panel. When you came here on your elective last year, you really impressed my staff, and I know that you would be very welcome once you've completed your residency. I have to admit that I have been waiting for this day and will be so proud of us working together. I hope you don't think it was too presumptive of me, but I did talk to the head of our internal medicine service, and she is most interested in discussing one of our vacant hospitalist positions with Julie, as that is what Julie told me she was interested in the last time we met."

Michael finished talking, internally exuberant at the idea of his son and future daughter-in-law joining the medical center, but trying to control himself emotionally in front of Sam and keep the conversation as professional as possible.

Sam paused. He looked worried. His father's enthusiastic response and lack of understanding of his wishes and career plans were exactly what he had feared. Sam was not quite sure how to go on, and what his father's reaction might be to his and Julie's plans. Would he be upset? Would he be angry? How could he continue the conversation in a sensitive way that would not offend his father?

In the ensuing silence, Michael couldn't wait for a response and decided to prompt his son. "Go on, Sam. Tell me what you think of this proposal. I think this will all work out really well. I do hope I haven't been inappropriate mentioning Julie to Dr. Lightfoot. I'm sorry if you think that. I've never intended to push you too much."

Michael suddenly started to worry at Sam's absent response and the look of uncertainty on his face. What if he had misjudged Sam's wishes? He knew he had never been good at reading him and had only gotten to really know him well in the last 10 years since the divorce. Before that he was always working and absent from home—something he now greatly regretted, because he had really not helped raise Sam and his sister, Katherine, beyond providing a physical home and financial security. Angie had done all the loving part of child-rearing. Now he started to feel anxious. Surely Sam wanted the same as he did? He continued talking to Sam, but now in a somewhat flustered tone.

"You seem to be uncertain, and I'm not sure what your silence means. I do hope I haven't misjudged anything, but I can tell you're worried. What do you think of these ideas? Please don't worry. I'll be OK with whatever you say. I'll support you in whatever direction you decide to go."

Finally Sam responded, in the knowledge that this was going to be just as difficult as he and Julie had envisaged. He spoke carefully, trying to be as gentle as possible on his dad.

"Dad, please hear me out and don't interrupt me. This is really hard for me to say, although I know it'll be harder for you to hear. I'm well aware that what I am going to say is going to be a huge disappointment for you, but we have to talk it through. While we really appreciate your kindness and enthusiasm, what you suggest is just not going to work for us. We want to work closely together and certainly wish to stay in the city here, but we've decided to accept positions that we've been offered by United Hospital across town."

Michael sat back in his chair in surprise. This was the last thing he had expected. His son working at the "opposition" city hospital. The place that had been the major rival of his own institution for many years. Their primary competitor. How could this be?

Sam continued. "There are lots of reasons for this that we can discuss, and while at a personal level I would love to be able to work with you, I just don't want to take a job in your medical center, and neither does Julie. Doing my elective there last year was busy and interesting, but frankly it put me off from taking a long-term job in the hospital. This is something that Julie and I have discussed at length, and we're making our own decisions, having thought about both of our career options at great length. I'm so sorry. I know you'll be very disappointed, but perhaps we can discuss some of the reasons so that you can understand better, because our minds are made up and we've already accepted our job offers and start on July 1st."

Michael tried to keep calm, even though he felt like much of his world had just fallen down around him. He took a long drink of his ice tea, now avoiding looking at Sam, and keeping his eyes on the rapidly darkening horizon. His mind scrambled for some consolation, and he quickly realized that at least Sam and Julie would be living close by, even if not working with him. It could have been worse. They could have decided to settle in a different city, or even in another state.

"Well, I didn't expect that. You're right," Michael said. "I know I have always somehow believed we would end up working together, especially when you chose emergency medicine as your residency. But at least you will both be close by and will be living locally so that you can both keep up with your running and hiking and all your outdoor interests."

"Yes, Dad, that's true. We love this area and all the sporting activities that are available for us to do. We're already mapping out our training schedules to do a marathon at the end of this year with Mark and Janice. You remember meeting them last August when we all went sailing together? They recently moved here and are now our closest friends, so we'll probably start looking for a home reasonably close to them on the other side of the city near United Hospital, where they also work."

"I know that you love all your outdoor activities, and with you and Julie both presumably doing shift work in hospitals, you'll have similar amounts of free time, so what I don't understand is why you've chosen to accept jobs at United, and not at the Medical Center. I know we are much more traditional in our ways, but we have a good name and pay better salaries," Michael concluded.

Sam looked up at his father, knowing that the next part of the conversation was going to be difficult. "Dad, I really respect all that you've done as a physician, and in the last decade, when we've been able to spend more time together, I've grown to love you a lot, but we both know it hasn't always been like this. The bottom line for me, Dad, is that I don't want to have the sort of life that you've had, even though we'll both be working the same job. And I'm afraid if I come to work with you at the, in my opinion, rather old-fashioned medical center, with its constant medical recruitment problems and its reputation for burning out physicians, I might end up like you were for many years before Mom finally walked out. I love Julie too much and I'm not prepared to risk that. And we want a better lifestyle than you had."

Michael looked rather taken aback and responded, "I thought that was all water under the bridge? I agree that I worked too hard, for too many hours, for years on end during your childhood, and that it was a major cause of my breakup with your mom, but that workstyle is not unusual for physicians. It was the norm in my day, and even now it is common, as you know. I'm a bit surprised that your fear of repeating my lifestyle is driving your work decisions."

Sam could see that his dad was still denying the impact his lack of work-life balance had had on him, and decided to gently expand his explanation and his fear of ending up like his father.

"OK, Dad. I guess I need to be completely straight with you. I know that you and Mom have always hidden a lot from Katherine and myself and tried to keep us sheltered from the sort of stresses you've both been through, and we really appreciate that. However, I found out a surprising amount about you from some of your colleagues at work when I was doing that elective in your department last year. I've since had a couple of long conversations with Mom to try and fill in the pieces, so that I could finally work out what was going on with you when I was a teenager. I've been blown away with what happened to you and wish you had told me yourself, but I guess you didn't want to because of the stigma and shame surrounding suicide attempts."

Michael sat up in surprise. How on earth could Sam have discovered his most painful secret? How did people in his workplace know what had happened more than a decade ago? He thought it was all behind him. Something in his past that he could now ignore.

"I can't believe you've found this out. I'm so sorry. I don't know what you must think of me. What a failure I was," he responded.

"If you found out about it from others, can I at least explain what happened from my perspective?" Michael continued. Sam nodded in reply.

Michael continued hesitantly. "I can tell you all the details later on if you wish, but in short I was working ridiculous hours because we were three physicians short in the department. I was almost never home, as you probably remember, and ended up having constant fights with your mom, so that I think I literally hid at work for 6 months at least to avoid that conflict. I started drinking to help me get to sleep and became irritable and depressed, but didn't recognize any of this myself, even though Angie tried to tell me how much I had changed. I started making mistakes at work and had my first-ever bad annual review from my chair, so I started to lose confidence in my clinical skills and found that I was taking longer and longer to see patients, checking and double-checking everything I did. In the end, following two more clinical errors, I was reprimanded by my departmental chair and sent home on administrative leave for two weeks. I was told that if I didn't improve my work I would likely be reported to the medical board. The thought of losing my medical license, and potentially my job, knowing that I had already probably lost my marriage and all my other prior interests, was just too much for me. I decided that you and Katherine would be better off without me because I was convinced I was such a failure. In retrospect, I can see I was also paranoid and possibly psychotic as a result of what I now know was my depressive illness. Over the month before I was sent home, I had gradually become convinced that there was a plot going on to destroy me led by my chair and that being sent home was proof of this. I believed that the only way out of my situation was to kill myself in an obvious way, hence, I felt, protecting others from being murdered along with me. I know it makes no sense, but I was really sick at the time. The irony of my situation is that it was my chair who saved my life. He was so concerned about me that he sent the police to my home to do a safety check, and they broke in to find me unconscious after I had taken a massive overdose. I was medically treated and put on a hold and sent to the local psychiatric unit, where I spent several weeks. Since then, until just a couple of years ago, I've had regular psychiatric follow-up, and even now I continue to take meds to prevent my recurrent depressive illness from occurring again."

Sam continued. "Dad, thank you for telling me this. I'll have lots more questions later I am sure. Just remember that I don't think you're a failure to have gone through this. You were sick with an illness just like any other illness. Physicians are like other people and are just as susceptible—or perhaps more so given the stresses on them—to having psychiatric disorders. We actually had a specific training course on physician health and well-being during my residency, so I learned a lot about this. I just had no idea until recently what had been going on. I simply knew that you were stressed and anxious and took some time off work when I was in middle school. I remember that time very well because I saw you at home a lot more than usual, which was great, and you were able to come and watch me play basketball, which you didn't normally do because you were always working. But I didn't know about your suicide attempt and how you nearly killed yourself. I know there's more than you've told me so far because Mom said you have had several depressive illnesses in your life and have recovered from them and kept on working even though it has been terribly hard for you, and of course for her. I never understood why you and Mom divorced, not until recently. I knew you weren't happy, but I didn't know why. By the way I still think you and Mom were perfect for each other, but I think she was sort of lonely at times because you were never home and when you were home you seemed so distant to all of us. Like you were lost in your head and unable to leave the hospital. Constantly thinking of work and your patients and never being able to separate from them and be with us."

Sam paused for a moment, knowing this whole conversation must be hard for his dad, and then continued. "So the single major reason for going to United Hospital is that I've been thinking a lot about what you went through, especially now that I know that I may be genetically vulnerable to developing depression myself. I'm determined not to replicate your mistakes. United seems much more concerned about their physicians' health and has an active program, run with strong support from their senior administrators, to support the well-being of their physician group, which your hospital still doesn't have, despite some of the efforts that I know you have made in your own department. Why do you think United is able to recruit and retain physicians and your hospital is not? At the end of the day, Julie and I want to have a family. We want to be able to be home with our children. We want to keep up our outside activities. And we want an interesting and rewarding job that's not overwhelming. We don't want to be seen as medical martyrs to a profession that drains us constantly, although we're prepared to work hard, but only to an extent, and not to a level that's harmful to us."

Sam stopped and took a breath. Calming himself down and wanting to make sure he didn't sound angry or disappointed in his dad, but genuinely wanting to uncover more of what had happened, and to learn from him.

"Given what Mom has told me about what happened to you, I do really want to talk with you more about what you did to survive, to not give in to the stress of the job, and to eventually flourish in your current job as chair of the department. I know I can learn a great deal from you—from what I see as your mistakes, I guess—and want to make sure that Julie and I don't end up like you and Mom, two lovely people who were separated by a difficult workstyle."

Throughout Sam's monologue, delivered with what seemed to be a combination of pent-up anxiety and intense passion, Michael had listened carefully, although a thousand thoughts had been flying through his mind. Was digging into such private and somewhat embarrassing parts of his life a good idea for either of them? Had he been right to hide the details of what he had gone through from Sam and Katherine? Should he have told him about the trauma and pain, or had he been right to deliberately try to protect his son and daughter? What really was his professional reputation—after all, suicide attempts were still highly stigmatized—if some people in his department knew what had happened? Could this process of sharing the truth of what he saw as his own failures turn into a positive revelation for Sam? His mind was spinning with uncertainty until he glanced upon his son's loving and respectful face, partly covered by shadows from the lengthening night. He had to trust Sam and knew he truly wanted to do the right thing to help him in any way he could.

"Well, Sam. You certainly have the ability to surprise me still. I would never have dreamed of you doing what you're suggesting and for the reasons you give, but I can certainly see that you've been doing a lot of thinking, more than I did at your age. You're making me reflect on some difficult things I've gone through and pushed deep inside me for many years. Somehow I feel a little relieved that you know. It's always been a bit odd knowing that I had such painful and difficult times and not being honest with you about them, when you were going into the same profession, and even the same medical discipline. I'm OK talking to you in more detail about what went on back then, but it's difficult."

"Sure, Dad. I'm just pleased we have this issue out in the open in our relationship. I'm certainly not going to be going out there telling anyone else. As far as I know, only Mom, Katherine, and Julie know any details. I'm just so pleased that you're prepared to talk about it and that you seem to have put that behind you now, because it explains a lot about why you do what you're doing now in your own workplace, even though I know you don't have a lot of support from your hospital hierarchy, who don't seem to understand the importance of protecting their most valuable asset—their physicians."

Sam poured two fresh glasses of iced tea and sat down across from his father, anxious to find out more from his father about how he had gradually changed his approach to medicine, and why.

He continued talking. "I don't know if you realize it, but I got to hear a great deal about you and your efforts to help all your staff while I was working in the ED last year. I heard how over the past 5 years, since you became chair, you have greatly improved the work environment for everyone. After all, everyone knows that EDs usually are the most stressful of any of the medical environments to work in. So many emergencies and life-and-death decisions. Throughout my residency I've been amazed at the number of patients who are angry, rude, and disrespectful. I know they were all in pain and distressed, but it astonishes me how much emotion the ED staff have to tolerate from the public. It's just not something that you think about until you've been there, but it makes sense. What your staff, especially some of the junior attending physicians, said to me regularly is that the thing they all admire you most for is the focus on physician and staff well-being that you've brought to your department despite how difficult it is for you to keep it going. Several times when I worked there they told me stories of how supported they felt by you and how great it was to be on your team. Several staff told me how awful it was before you became chair. They really appreciate the changes you've made. They told me how you would come by at all hours of the day and night to check on them and on how they were managing. They said the way you implemented a new backup schedule so physicians can take time off without guilt for their own sick days or emergencies has helped morale a lot. They're also aware that you take all sorts of actions to support them in a difficult hospital workplace environment where they say they feel the hospital administration is primarily interested in keeping them as busy and productive as possible."

Michael looked a bit embarrassed and turned away from his son, sort of uncomfortable hearing these compliments, although concerned to hear about the adverse perception of the hospital leadership.

"Thanks, Sam. It's really good to know the well-being program changes I've made in the department are appreciated. For me that's the single most important part of my job as departmental chair. I'm pleased that they told you all this. Were there any specific stories or interventions that they described that you remember, because they might be pointers for me for the future?"

Sam thought for a minute before responding. "Yes, there were a few. The innovation that they really respect you for most, and that stood out to me, was actually the introduction of scribes for the EMR. I was told numerous times by your physicians that their lives were radically changed by the introduction of scribes into the ED, and how you had led a huge fight with the hospital administration to get them. They said that before scribes were introduced, they had to write all their own notes in the EMR [electronic medical record] and that in the rush and hurry of the ED this was almost impossible. They ended up writing notes at home, after shifts and in their own time, and trying to keep up with EMRs in that environment had just been frustrating and exhausting. They told me how the hospital tried to make the doctors use templates, all sorts of recording systems and extra documentation training, and the doctors tried these approaches but to no avail. They said that when the EMR was introduced, the hospital hierarchy was rigid about insisting that all clinical staff in all departments use it, and administration was really not interested in listening to their complaints about how much time it added to the consultation, or whether the demands of one department were greater than others. The physicians told me that for the first 5 years of the EMR all that happened was that they were constantly behind with their notes, and they stopped enjoying seeing patients because there was just this huge load of documentation required to satisfy all the diverse groups of people who wanted more and more data to be collected in the EMR. I don't know if you fully realize the impact that lessening the burden of the EMR has had, but it seems to me that it has been huge for how the physicians feel about their workload, and it has dramatically improved their lifestyle because they no longer have to constantly catch up with notes. So let me turn this around, Dad, because this is one of the topics I want to understand. I would love to know from you, how did you get the idea for scribes, and how on earth did you get them introduced in your own department, especially since the hospital administration was so against the idea?"

Michael replied quickly and enthusiastically, feeling on fairly safe ground here. "And you know, they're still very much against scribes, so mine is still the only department that has them. There were both personal and practical departmental reasons for arguing for the need for them, and I felt very strongly about this. The EMR was introduced in our hospital about 7 years ago, just before I became chair, and I had to go and learn how to use it just like all my colleagues. As someone in my late 40s at the time, this was a steep learning curve. I literally learned to touch-type and took evening classes to master that skill because I was determined not to be one of those awful "two-fingered typists" that you still see occasionally in the group of elder physicians. I soon realized that I was taking a lot more time to do my notes, and I started literally timing myself, even though my typing was good. I tried automated dictating, but there were too many errors that took too long to correct, and I realized early on that using the EMR simply took more time than paper records, mainly because of the extra data demands and time to log on and click through the software—turning pages in a paper record is much quicker. All the doctors were upset with how difficult it was to use the EMR and how much time it took. To cut a long story short, I became interested in this whole issue and did a lot of research on it, and discovered that the single intervention that seemed to work best was scribes. These are typically bright young students, often premed, who want to get experience seeing patients and working in clinical settings and who usually volunteer for these roles in droves wherever there is a medical school. So from then on it was just a matter of convincing the hospital administration. I did economic and workflow studies of how much time would be saved by my physicians, and consequently how many more patients per shift they could see, and connected with the university pre-med program. Eventually I was successful in getting agreement to fund a pilot program. This worked well, and the rest is history. And you're right, I do get lots of kudos for this from my staff, who have seen an immediate benefit in terms of their well-being and lifestyle. I'm not suggesting this is the perfect answer for all departments, because the presence of scribes can be intrusive, as you know, especially when consultations become very emotional or if the patient objects to their presence. But solving the EMR time problem is one of the best ways of supporting physician well-being. I just wish there were more things I could implement as successfully as this, but change is a constant battle in my hospital, as it seems you've realized."

"Dad, that is a great achievement, but there must have been other reasons you went down that path. It sounds like it took a huge amount of time and energy. Were there are other reasons?" Sam asked.

"Sam, you're obviously already a great doctor. You're so perceptive. Of course there were. One of the things you find in medicine is that you're sometimes heavily influenced by certain cases that you see. I told you that I saw the EMR as a stressor and was pleased I hadn't had to deal with it when I was depressed and tried to kill myself. Well, the final straw for me that made me determined to reduce this stress on all of us physicians in the ED came a few months after I was made chair. I was in the ED one evening on a routine shift. As you know, I continue two shifts a week even now to make sure that, despite my administrative load, I still have my finger on the clinical pulse of the department, and to demonstrate to my staff that I, as the leader, still work with patients like they do. Well, the case that was my tipping point on this issue was a physician suicide. I will never forget this patient. He was about 40, a primary care physician at a different health system, and he was brought in after taking a massive overdose from which he simply never recovered. He died in our ICU 2 days after admission. I never had a chance to speak with him, my patient, because he was unconscious, but I did talk extensively to his wife and children. They described his life and told me about the increasing number of hours of medical record documentation he was doing at home as he tried to get on top of a newly introduced EMR system and still maintain seeing the same number of patients per day. His wife was just so angry and described herself as a long-standing "EMR widow." She told me how she had been trying to persuade him to change jobs and to move to a clinic with paper records so they could have their life back. He refused and was determined to keep up with his colleagues and not look like a failure when the weekly data on note completions were sent out to everyone. But each week when he had the most notes incomplete was a source of professional humiliation and stress for him. It was evident to me that she didn't realize the seriousness of his overdose and the lethal concoction of drugs that he had taken.

"While I was talking to her, I just kept having flashbacks to my own suicide attempt and thought about how similar this physician was to me. How I had been given a second chance, and he was probably not going to get one. To me it was obvious that while the stresses on both of us were different, he was the victim of at least some pressures that we could work on and modify. So yes, you're right, there was another reason. And you know what I did? I made a copy of the notes I made on that physician and, after deleting his name and identifiers, kept them on me in my lab coat pocket at all times until I got the scribes, as a constant reminder of why I had to make this change. You know, I still think of his wife sometimes, even now, and of his two young and very confused sons who have had to grow up without their father. It's so ironic that the introduction of the EMR, which most physicians strongly support for patient care, is often associated for many doctors with the unintended consequence of increased stress, more time spent on notation, and less direct time with patients."

Michael sat back further in his chair. He had never told anyone this story and had never even admitted out loud the parallels he had drawn with his own suicide attempt, although he had often thought about them. This was a story he had not even told the therapist he used to see because he felt that this physician had probably been suffering for a long time and either no one noticed or, if they had, his situation had been ignored. His death had surely been preventable. Someone must have seen that he was not doing well. He waited for Sam's response, which came after a short silence.

"Dad, I'm so sorry. I can see how stressful that must have been for you. And how it must have made you reflect on your own situation. And probably on your marriage to Mom, which clearly became a casualty of your work. What an impact a suicide must have on the families. His poor wife and their children. And how awful his friends and colleagues must have felt. I can see why you and Mom kept your difficulties secret from Katherine and me at the time. I guess I've been lucky and none of my medical friends have attempted suicide, although several have seen psychiatrists and counselors and have usually found that helpful. I think my generation is rather different from yours and is more prepared to seek help if we get stressed. Also, we did get some education on physician health both as medical students and in residency, and I understand your generation of physicians did not. I'm glad we haven't been left to struggle on in silence like you had to, but as you can see this is one of the reasons driving my and Julie's decisions to work at a place that is more supportive of our work-life balance. Having said all that, it's great that you've taken action to reduce the chance that your own staff will get into his situation even if you cannot affect the whole hospital."

"That's true. I'm very aware of that, and it really worries me that other physicians in my health system may be at risk. The EMR is not the only stressor. There are other issues that physicians deal with every day. When you did your elective last year, did you get told about some of the other things we've introduced to help not just my ED physicians but all our ED staff?" Michael asked.

Sam replied, "I guess you mean things like the regular departmental trips to the soccer and basketball games? And the internal competitions and spot awards? One of the physicians told me about the way you encourage what he called "random acts of kindness" to patients and staff, and how you've arranged for gifts and boxes of fruit to be available to be given out whenever someone has done something great. They think it's really cool and feel proud to be in a department that does that."

"You're right. But I try and encourage a lot more than that. To prevent burnout, depression, and substance use, I've really worked hard to introduce a whole series of initiatives, led by an enthusiastic young attending who we've given the title "Director of ED Well-Being." She is amazing and organizes all sorts of activities to engage the staff and boost their morale, so that they can help themselves as much as possible and strengthen their personal resilience. There's research coming out now that demonstrates that it's necessary to make both individual and organizational changes to really reduce the impact of the fairly stressful and toxic work environment that can occur in today's hospitals. So while she focuses mainly on helping staff cope better, at the same time I have changed our management process and really gotten as many people as possible involved in departmental decision making so that they know they are listened to and are more in control of their workplace. We've been experimenting with some different patient workflows recently, for instance, that seem to be much more efficient at reducing our wait times, while at the same time getting patients admitted more quickly. The input from staff is quite valuable. They frequently bring fresh ideas that improve morale and more often than not end up also improving efficiencies across our department."

Sam was listening intently. "That's amazing, Dad. I actually didn't realize you were doing so much to support all your staff. It sounds like you've made a lot of changes in the last year since I was there. I admire how you must be taking on the culture of medicine at your hospital with your changes. I see the attendings I work for commonly being emotionally constrained by the need to appear independent and strong. They see weakness or asking for help as a sign of failure, instead of being able to acknowledge that it's a normal reflection of a high-pressure occupation being carried out by people who are all human and have the full range of human strengths and frailties. There is a huge deficit in medical education on this topic, and I know that in your hospital there is no effective physician well-being committee and little attempt by the administration to support physicians, beyond what you're doing in your own department."

Michael replied, "I appreciate your thoughts, Sam, but the problem is wider than that. You know it's still common at some medical schools for students to go and get drunk as a way of celebrating after exams. Every year at many schools one or more students or residents get DUIs after such celebrations. I actually heard this happened to one of our medical residents recently, when they drunk-drove after a hospital party celebrating the end of the first year of residency."

"That's awful," said Sam in surprise. "What a dreadful paradox. Making yourself sick and endangering your career as a response to passing an exam. It makes no sense. I heard that used to happen years ago but didn't realize it was still common."

Michael continued. "It's true and sad. There is still almost no education on physician well-being at the medical school that sends students to my hospital, beyond a few lectures on the importance of avoiding drugs and alcohol, whereas in my view it should be a core part of the curriculum. As I've told you, I was almost one of those 400 doctors per year who die by suicide. Do you realize that's the equivalent of two large medical school classes every year dying like that? Never mind all the other physicians with untreated illnesses. We desperately need to do more education on the issue, as well as change the way we work. After all, what use is a car if you don't regularly service it and look after it properly? It seems so odd to me that we don't do that for ourselves as a profession. I am pleased that your generation is doing better than mine and that the choices you and Julie are making are starting to make a lot of sense to me, as it's clear you are thinking about how to look after yourselves properly."

Sam responded eagerly. "I haven't mentioned this before, Dad, but one of the reasons I've chosen to go to United Hospital is that they've offered me the chance to teach and supervise their medical students and residents on the topic of physician health. So I plan on including all the issues we've been discussing in the curriculum I need to develop, but I also want to include the importance of physical fitness, good sleep, and keeping up relationships and interests, as well as other lifestyle issues.

Sam looked up at his father listening attentively and continued on enthusiastically. "The other exciting innovation that United is introducing is the implementation of the Institute for HealthCare Improvement framework to allow physicians and other clinical staff to find more joy in work. I know that the term "joy in work" sounds a bit hokey, but I've read about the program and it sounds really good. The aim is to ask staff what matters most to them and to particularly to identify any local impediments to finding joy in the workplace, and then the organization commits to a systems-based approach, using improvement science methods, to improve everyone's situation, taking the view that making joy in work is a shared responsibility at all levels of the organization. You know, despite all the good things we can do for ourselves as individuals, what I've found out in my experience is that in complicated systems like hospitals, you can't just "resilience yourself" out of burnout or stress—you primarily need a whole-scale organizational approach. And that is where United is so far ahead of the Medical Center. It will be exciting to be part of this new way of working."

"That sounds fascinating. I will look up that program. I hadn't heard about it," replied Michael

Sam continued more slowly and thoughtfully, pleased he seemed to have his father's full attention and interest. "Talking to you about this is really helpful, but given your personal experiences and your long-standing interest in this whole area, I'd like to know if there any really big barriers or changes that you can see that I need to think about. They may be issues I might have to mention, just to show I am aware of them, even if they cannot easily be changed in the short run."

Michael sat back and thought, before replying, speaking in a careful and deliberate way. "You know, unfortunately, I think there are still going to be three major barriers for medical students and residents, even if everything else is improved, and I'm really not sure how you get over these. None of them are realistically going to change soon."

"Such as?" asked Sam.

"Well, the first is the enduring professional attitudes that require extraordinary levels and hours of work from medical school onwards, and the consequence of constantly having to delay gratification because there's always another goal to achieve before reward. The work hours of residents are an example there—as you know from your own experience, they are constantly being modified and it's very hard to have all programs comply with them, so many residents still work more hours than they should be doing. But this is a difficult issue because the only way to get experience is to do the work. So I'm not sure what the answer is to that, although some countries have solved this issue and have restricted resident work hours more successfully. Maybe you could also do some research on that?"

Michael stopped and took a sip of his drink before continuing. "The other two issues are easier to solve, and I sincerely hope they will be addressed over time. The first is the dreadful way medical student board exams are scored in a numeric competitive way, the scores of which have become way too important in determining whether you get into residency. You experienced this yourself when you had to apply for a popular residency like emergency medicine. Medical students with low scores on their boards don't even get an interview. This just means that medical students are forced to dramatically overwork to get high scores, rather than simply prove that they are competent and are fit to practice.

"You're right Dad," Tom replied. "I can remember the anxiety we all had taking our medical school steps and aiming not just to pass, which is all we should have been required to do, but to get as high a score as possible. I can remember thinking I had effectively failed when I only scored in the top 20% of students nationally because I knew that that score might affect my residency choice. It's completely ridiculous when you think about it rationally. What is the final issue that you think needs changing?"

"The second issue concerns the excessive fees you have to pay, and how they burden students and residents and frequently affect their career decision making. There is no time to do paid work at medical school as there is if you are doing a PhD, and this debt is driving medical students into high-paying specialties like radiology, ophthalmology, and dermatology, and creating shortages in areas like primary care, pediatrics, and family medicine where we desperately need more doctors. As we know, I have done my best to help you financially so that you only have a small debt, but from what you say Julie was not so lucky, and it's awful that she's saddled with close to the average medical student debt of $170,000. I know that this must have been part of your decision to go to United Health, since they're known to pay a signing-on bonus, and hope you've negotiated this so you can pay down your debt somewhat. I was talking to a married pair of residents at work the other day who are about to take up junior attending jobs in our hospital, and between them they owe over $400,000. And this is at a time in their lives when they should be trying to buy a house and start a family. It's just so difficult. That has to change somehow because it puts young doctors like you and Julie under huge financial pressure and does drive your career decisions."

"Well, Dad, you've hit the nail on the head. You'll be glad to hear that we do both have signing-on bonuses, and we're also being given cheap loans to buy a home, although these extras are a bit like golden handcuffs, since we only keep them as long as we stay for at least 5 years. They do make a big difference, though, and will allow us to be much more independent and to have more control over our careers and our lives than you have had at times."

"Talking of more control," said Michael, "I need you to teach me how to make that amazing barbecue sauce you said you were planning to use on our steaks. Let's get going on that. I bought all the ingredients you emailed me and want to understand why it is so complicated. I can't believe you need apple cider vinegar, Worcester sauce, ketchup, brown and white sugar, peppers, lemon juice, onion powder and ground mustard seeds just for a sauce. It's very different from buying something premade as I've always done."

Commentary

This scenario focuses on a range of solutions that are all perfectly possible, and which will reduce the number of physician suicides, as discussed in detail in Chapter 1, as well as the stressors on doctors more generally. We all know that prevention is better than cure, and this is the approach that the medical profession should be taking. So when Sam is putting together his curriculum on physician health for medical students and residents, what are the sort of preventive activities he should be thinking about discussing that will hopefully be introduced during their upcoming medical careers?

The first is obviously education and research about the problem. After all, if you don't know about an issue, how can you address it? This is starting to happen mainly at a graduate level post medical school, but today's attempts at self-education within the profession are vestigial at best and primarily involve five sets of activities, all of which have been highlighted in previous chapters and are outlined below:

1. The existence of physician health programs in almost all states, and medical staff well-being committees nationally, as discussed in Chapter 9, both of which have primarily clinical and educational mandates as described on the Federation of State Physician Health Programs Web site (https://www.fsphp.org).

2. A series of conferences that have been held, in some cases for more than 30 years and with an increasingly larger network of physicians and

other healthcare professionals who are interested and expert in the topic. In the past 10 years, such conferences have become increasingly common and larger, with the most popular one being the biannual International Conference on Physician Health, a collaborative meeting sponsored by the American Medical Association (AMA), the Canadian Medical Association, and the British Medical Association (https://www.ama-assn.org/events/international-conference-physician-health). The 2017 American Conference on Physician Health in San Francisco was sold out within weeks of the conference announcement.

3. An increasingly strong research and education literature that is gradually developing. Most key references are given throughout this book in the relevant chapters. The American Medical Association has been exceptional in its leadership and production of a series of four first-class educational products that are available free online (American Medical Association 2018a, 2018b, 2018c, 2018d) and is currently developing wellness competencies for education programs. The National Academy of Medicine Action Collaborative on Clinician Well-being and Resilience (https://nam.edu/initiatives/clinician-resilience-and-well-being) is another excellent recent innovation that has a strong educational and culture change management approach. It includes five workgroups that are focused on research, on data and metrics, on conceptual models, on external factors and workflows, and on messaging and communications issues, as well as a very creative group concentrating on publications and art of relevance to clinician health and well-being. Sam, in the scenario, mentioned the Institute for Healthcare Improvement Framework for Improving Joy in Work (Perlo et al. 2017), which is an excellent white paper that is intended to guide health care organizations in a participative process to enable leaders to better understand the barriers to joy in work and to create and leverage strategies to address these issues. Several of the professional organizations apart from the AMA have also set up Web sites with helpful information for their members, notably the American Psychiatric Association (https://www.psychiatry.org/psychiatrists/practice/well-being-and-burnout), American Society of Addiction Medicine (https://www.asam.org/advocacy/issues), and the American Academy of Family Practitioners (https://www.aafp.org/news/focus-on-physician-well-being.html) among others. Several multidisciplinary research groups have developed in the past decade and have started to focus on this area, notably at the Mayo Clinic (http://www.mayo.edu/research/centers-programs/physician-well-being-program/) and Stanford (https://wellmd.stanford.edu/), although grants for work in this area are still few in number and hard to obtain.

4. The existence of many physicians who treat other physicians and who, for clinical purposes, have become interested and knowledgeable about the area.

5. The recent, and much needed, interest by the Accreditation Council for Graduate Medical Education (ACGME; http://www.acgme.org/What-We-Do/Initiatives/Physician-Well-Being), which has mandated education about physician health to commence in all residency programs nationally, commencing July 2017. This excellent start to universal medical education on physician health focuses on the topic primarily as a professionalism and patient safety issue. This initiative should lead to all residents within the next few years being taught both factual content about physician health, as highlighted in this book, and some essential skills, such as how to approach a colleague who appears to be unwell, or who is practicing in an unsafe manner.

This, then, is the current broad baseline of physician health and well-being activities that reaches most physicians nationally at some level, but that also misses the majority of the 50% of all physicians who work in small private practices, as described in Chapter 9, and most medical students and residents.

What needs to happen next is the gradual spread, expansion, and dissemination of all of these activities much more widely and deeply with the aim of eventually changing the culture of medical practice. There is an almost complete lack of formal educational curricula or courses on physician health and resilience training in medical schools and a need for self-care competencies to be integrated into the medical school curricula nationally by the Association of American Medical Colleges, perhaps working with the AMA, which has taken a lead in this area. Of equal importance is the development of formal curricula to support the ACGME requirements, with courses and resources then being developed using the principles of adult education, such as the inclusion of case-based interactive learning, that can be widely used nationally and internationally. These educational programs for medical students and residents should, of course, also be developed further to apply to postgraduate physicians out in practice to meet the current increasing need for this topic.

A second important educational need that has not currently been met, and which is highlighted in Chapters 4 and 8, is the need for courses and curricula designed to teach physicians how to treat other physicians, as well as other VIPs or challenging patients.

Resilience, as discussed in Chapter 2, is the ability of a person to maintain social and personal stability in the face of adversity. Importantly, the capacity for resilience can be taught, and it's well known that such interventions can improve patient care practices. Beresin et al. (2016) have examined the need for resilience education and training in medical school, during residency, and all life long. They noted the following broad factors as contributing to physician distress:

- Shortages of health care professionals
- Demanding caseloads
- Verbal abuse and other belittling or bullying behavior
- Tremendous debt following lengthy medical education
- Increased regulatory pressures
- Decreased insurance reimbursements for services
- Staying current with overwhelming amounts of new knowledge

They commented that these challenges "are compounded by our profession's hidden curriculum—the reluctance to admit weakness, to expose our shame of suffering from a psychiatric disorder, or even discuss the pressures we share" (p. 9).

It's possible to overcome such issues, however, and Beresin et al. (2016) reviewed a number of studies of programs that have led to increased physician and student resilience as examples of the sorts of interventions that could be introduced more widely. One such intervention, from a study at the Mayo Clinic (West et al. 2014), consisted of several months of biweekly facilitated discussion groups incorporating mindfulness and shared learning experiences in protected paid time, while another study of brief online cognitive-behavioral therapy showed a reduction in the likelihood of suicidal ideation in interns (Guille et al. 2015) Several other initiatives in different states are highlighted in a short but useful online Medscape Continuing Medical Education course on fighting physician burnout (Sara 2018).

Beresin et al. (2016) laid out a number of components of what could become a core curriculum for medical students and residents that might act as a self-care toolkit to be used throughout their careers. A more comprehensive curriculum, which includes some of their suggestions and ideas taken from the cases in this book, might be as follows:

- Regular participation in process-oriented reflective small groups
- Mentoring and mentee supervision opportunities
- Decision making and clinical reasoning that take into account future changes in medicine, such as the increasing number of data sources and artificial intelligence algorithms to be understood that are increas-

ingly making physicians both data analysts who are expert in pattern matching and diagnosticians

- Content on the various specific psychiatric, substance use, and personality disorders described in this book that affect physicians, and how to recognize and treat them in any physician, including the individuals themselves
- Curricular content on personal identity development and transformation, the interaction between burnout and physician health (including suicidality), empathy, compassion, resiliency, and how to become reflective practitioners
- Modules and active participation and learning about mindfulness, exercise, nutrition, and relationships
- Learning about systems interactions, institutional awareness, and resources that can be used to enhance physician well-being
- Specific skills development in interpersonal professional relationships
- Modules and discussion groups on financial and business skills
- Leadership and media training
- Creation of opportunities to strengthen professional and social relationships and how to network widely and appropriately

Going beyond the formal educational side, Sam could focus on himself as an example for his future student and physician colleagues and mention his understanding of how to maintain his own health, increase his personal resilience, and maintain his long-term pride and joy at being able to have one of the most meaningful careers possible, as a practicing physician. This involves being constantly aware of a number of lifestyle and personal developmental issues as described in the literature and throughout this book.

The first cornerstone for well-being is the maintenance of a balanced life. There's nothing wrong with working hard, and for long hours, as long as there is a balance between work, relationships, and other interests and pursuits. Working hard and playing hard is fine, but working hard and doing nothing else is a prescription for disaster, as described by Sam's father in the scenario. Doing the Well-Being Index developed by the Mayo Clinic research team (www,mywellbeingindex.org), as discussed in Chapter 2, is a good way for individuals to self-assess. Norcross (2017) has described the importance of balance in the life of a physician, demonstrating how many physicians have excessive imbalances, with too much time and effort devoted to work. Balance means paying attention to relationships, families, and friendships; getting exercise; taking holidays; and having hobbies and interests outside of medicine; as well as maintaining spiritual

perspectives and beliefs. While the long-standing medical practice of delayed gratification is, at exam time, inevitable, self-rewards and positive
reinforcements deliberately planned into any schedule can still make a big
difference.

There are a number of very simple practical things that Sam could promote to his students, including setting themselves a broad personal goal,
such as to flourish, have peak experiences, and share them. Such personal
goals are very important, and Sam may find it helpful to have his students
write their goals in capital letters in a prominent place where they spend
time to constantly remind themselves of the importance of this objective.

Strategies that are known to be helpful for Sam to describe include exploring and finding meaning in work, deliberately seeking out humor and
cultivating the positives in his life, making time for play, and celebrating
the successes of himself and others. Equally importantly, taking time for
family and friends—and specifically cultivating and maintaining friendships and relationships—is vital, as is taking vacations. One very effective
way of improving relationships is to be a friend for others, to listen to
them and help as necessary, in the knowledge that what goes around will
come around. Regular exercise and a method to enable a daily release of
frustrations are also of key importance. This might be scheduling a gym,
yoga, or tai chi session; walking a dog; meditating mindfully; or just taking stairs and walking places rather than using elevators and cars—all of
which are easy long-term lifestyle adaptations. The restorative power of
sleep is also vital, so Sam should emphasize the importance of making
sure his students and residents sleep well and pay attention to their sleep-
wake cycle as much as possible. Planning time for regular study instead
of pulling all-night sessions prior to exams is healthy, just as is always ensuring that all doctors and students not only have a personal primary care
physician but regularly visit with this individual and have all the required
preventive physical examinations and labs done, rather than treating
themselves.

From an individual perspective Sam could talk about the importance
of mentoring, which, as a process, is of enormous importance and has
been shown by Straus et al. (2013) to be associated with much improved
personal and professional outcomes. In an interesting qualitative compar-
ative study of 54 faculty, these authors described successful mentoring relationships as being characterized by reciprocity, mutual respect, clear
expectations, personal connection, and shared values, and failed mentoring relationships as being characterized by poor communication, lack of
commitment, personality differences, perceived (or real) competition,
conflicts of interest, and the mentor's lack of experience. Many academic

programs either strongly encourage or mandate mentoring relationships for junior faculty, and similar programs have been developed in most medical schools, where senior students are routinely paired with juniors, but such relationships are much less common in private practice environments, especially in those that can be quite competitive, such as in the surgical and interventional specialties.

Finally, Sam could address the two practical and substantive causes of stress that all medical students remark on—namely, the continuing existence of competitive graded examinations, including the three United States Medical Licensing Examination (USMLE) Steps, and the financial burden and likely debt incurred through medical school.

Most students arrive at medical school with a supreme belief in their academic ability. They are used to being in the top few students in all classes they have taken, and many have not been seriously academically challenged previously. Suddenly they are in a class of 100–200 other similar students, and not only do many no longer stand out, there are a number who are initially shocked by the need to struggle to keep up with the really massive cognitive and academic load that is required. Although many medical schools examine students with internal results graded as pass/fail, which dramatically reduces the competitive component among the students, there remain many highly competitive elements to the medical school curriculum. The two main components are the process for the awarding of honors and the need not to just pass but to obtain very high scores on the national USMLE Boards, both of which are highly influential in determining success in getting into residency programs. The board exams are exhausting and stressful, and taking them requires much planning and thought. Sam could teach students how to work consistently for them, scheduling tests at a time that allows them to have a break afterward, and using the school's academic mentoring resources to learn the multiple-choice techniques involved, and practice by taking multiple practice tests, rather than doing last-minute "swotting."

Financial debt is the other major stressor for many students, and the potential extent of this debt may well determine which medical school an applicant goes to, as well as which residency program he or she enters. The Association of American Medical Colleges (2017) estimated that the average debt balance for 2017 graduates was $190,000. All medical schools offer financial aid to students, and counterintuitively the private schools not infrequently may sometimes end up being the cheapest option because of their massive endowments, compared with public schools. All students and doctors need to try to continuously reduce their long-term debt position and increase their own financial literacy, as recommended by Kaplan

Test Prep (2017). In this setting it is worrying that a national program that enables students to be relieved of their debt if they work in the public sector in specified positions (including time in residency) for 10 years after medical school graduation is currently under review and is not definitely being continued. Fortunately, there are some impressive financial guides available for students and residents, such as that available at the Student Loan Hero (2017) Web site, which Sam certainly needs to include in his teaching.

It's evident that more attention is being paid to the issue of physician health. In the scenario Sam quite correctly says that you cannot simply "resilience yourself" out of burnout. So while most of the interventions discussed in this chapter have applied to individuals, they need to be implemented within a health organization, such as the one preferred by Sam and Julie, where there are systemic changes occurring that support physician health and well-being, and the health and well-being of all other clinicians. In such organizations this will ultimately lead to a change in the culture of healthcare and, consequently, better overall patient care delivered by healthier and happier clinicians. Ultimately, over time this will reduce the unacceptably high levels of burnout, depression, anxiety, substance abuse, and suicide currently seen within the profession. It is also hoped that during Sam's career, over the next 30 years, this improvement will persist and that physicians of the future will be less likely to kill themselves than the present generation. Physicians of the future, such as Sam and Julie, do have an opportunity to live more balanced, rewarding lives with their partners and families than frequently happens now, and therefore be able to continue to practice excellent high-quality medicine while working in one of the most rewarding and meaningful professions imaginable.

References

American Medical Association: STEPS Forward. Improving physician resiliency. 2018a. Available at: https://www.stepsforward.org/modules/improving-physician-resilience. Accessed January 29, 2018.

American Medical Association: STEPS Forward. Physician wellness: preventing resident and fellow burnout. 2018b. Available at: https://www.stepsforward.org/modules/physician-wellness. Accessed January 29, 2018.

American Medical Association: STEPS Forward. Preventing physician burnout. 2018c. Available at: https://www.stepsforward.org/modules/physician-burnout. Accessed January 29, 2018.

American Medical Association: STEPS Forward. Preventing physician distress and suicide. 2018d. Available at: https://www.stepsforward.org/modules/preventing-physician-suicide. Accessed January 29, 2018.

Association of American Medical Colleges: Debt, costs and loan repayment fact card. October 2017. Available at: https://members.aamc.org/iweb/upload/ 2017%20Debt %20Fact%20Card.pdf.

Beresin EV, Milligan TA, Balon R, et al: Physician wellbeing: a critical deficiency in resilience education and training. Acad Psychiatry 40(1):9–12, 2016 26691141

Guille C, Zhao Z, Krystal J, et al: Web-based cognitive behavioral therapy intervention for the prevention of suicidal ideation in medical interns: a randomized clinical trial. JAMA Psychiatry 72(12):1192–1198, 2015

Kaplan Test Prep: The importance of financial literacy for pre-med students. July 14, 2017. Available at: https://www.kaptest.com/blog/med-school-pulse/ 2017/07/14/the-importance-of-financial-literacy-for-pre-med-students. Accessed January 29, 2018.

Norcross W: Physician stress and burnout. Paper presented at the Western States Regional Conference on Physicians' Well-Being, University of California, Riverside, May 24, 2017

Perlo J, Balik B, Swensen S, et al: IHI Framework for Improving Joy in Work. IHI White Paper. Cambridge, MA, Institute for Healthcare Improvement, 2017. Available at http://www.ihi.org/resources/Pages/IHIWhitePapers/Framework-Improving-Joy-in-Work.aspx.

Sara GA: Combating physician burnout: tactics and strategies for easing burnout. Medscape, 2018. Available at: https://www.medscape.com/courses/business/ 100012. Accessed January 29, 2018.

Straus SE, Johnson MO, Marquez C, et al: Characteristics of successful and failed mentoring relationships: qualitative study across 2 institutions. Acad Med 88(1):82–89, 2013 23165266

Student Loan Hero: The ultimate student loan repayment guide for doctors. January 21, 2017. Available at: https://studentloanhero.com/featured/ultimate-student-loan-repayment-guide-for-doctors. Accessed January 29, 2018.

West CP, Dyrbye LN, Rabatin JT, et al: Intervention to promote physician wellbeing, job satisfaction, and professionalism: a randomized clinical trial. JAMA Intern Med 174(4):527–533, 2014 24515493

Index

Page numbers printed in **boldface** type refer to tables and figures.